TOP 200

Other books by Ronald J. Tallarida

The Dose-Response Relation in Pharmacology
Ronald J. Tallarida and Leonard S. Jacob
New York, Springer-Verlag 1979

Manual of Pharmacologic Calculations with Computer Programs
Ronald J. Tallarida and Rodney B. Murray
New York, Springer-Verlag 1981

TOP 200
Revised and Updated

Ronald J. Tallarida, Ph.D.
Professor of Pharmacology
Temple University School of Medicine
Philadelphia, Pennsylvania

A compendium of pharmacologic and
therapeutic information on the most
widely prescribed drugs in America

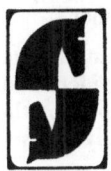

Springer-Verlag Berlin Heidelberg GmbH

Ronald J. Tallarida, Ph.D.
Professor of Pharmacology
Temple University School of Medicine
Philadelphia, Pennsylvania 19140 U.S.A.

Library of Congress Cataloging in Publication Data
Tallarida, Ronald J.
  Top 200.
  Includes bibliographies and index.
  1. Drugs—Handbooks, manuals, etc.   2. Drugs—
United States—Handbooks, manuals, etc.   I. Title.
[DNLM: 1. Drugs—Handbooks.   QV 772 T147t]
RM300.T32   1982   615'.1   82–10732

© 1982 by Springer-Verlag Berlin Heidelberg
Originally published by Springer-Verlag New York Inc. 1982

ISBN 978-1-4899-6748-0   ISBN 978-1-4899-6746-6 (eBook)
DOI 10.1007/978-1-4899-6746-6

9 8 7 6 5 4 3 2 1

To Theresa

Contents

Classification Based on Pharmacologic Action
and/or Therapeutic Use
Top 200 Drugs (year 1981)

AMEBICIDES & TRICHOMONACIDES
  Flagyl   114

ANALGESICS
Acetaminophen & Combinations
  Parafon Forte   235
  Phenaphen/Codeine   246
Aspirin & Combinations
  Equagesic   101
  Fiorinal   112
  Norgesic Forte   206
  Synalgos-DC   293
Narcotics & Combinations
  Fiorinal/Codeine   113
  Percodan   242
  Phenaphen/Codeine   246
  Synalgos-DC   293
  Tylenol/Codeine   326
Synthetics & Combinations
  Darvocet-N 100   71
  Darvon Compound 65   73
  Talwin   298
Urinary Tract
  Pyridium   265
Other
  Motrin   193
  Zomax   343

ANOREXICS (antiobesity)
  Fastin   110

Other
Meclomen   180
Motrin   193
Nalfon   198
Naprosyn   199
Tolectin DS   315

ANTINAUSEANTS
Antivert   23
Atarax   30
Bendectin   40
Compazine   61
Thorazine   305
Tigan   310
Vistaril   339

ANTIPARASITICS
Kwell   155

ANTI-PARKINSONISM DRUGS
Artane   28
Cogentin   58

ANTIPRURITICS
Atarax   30
Valisone   328

ANTIPSYCHOTICS
Compazine   61
Mellaril   183
Stelazine   285
Thorazine   305
Triavil   320

Generic Index

Acetaminophen
Darvocet-N 100   71
Parafon Forte   235
Phenaphen/Codeine   246
Tylenol/Codeine   326

ALCOHOL
Ambenyl Expectorant   12
Benylin Cough Syrup   43
Dimetane Expectorant   83
Phenergan Expectorant   248
Phenergan Expectorant/Codeine   250
Phenergan VC Expectorant   251
Phenergan VC Expectorant/Codeine   253

ALLUPURINOL
Zyloprim   344

AMINOPHYLLINE
Aminophylline   14

AMITRIPTYLINE HCL
Elavil   94
Generic   16
Limbitrol   168
Triavil   320

AMMONIUM CHLORIDE
Ambenyl Expectorant   12

AMOXICILLIN
Amoxicillin   18

Top 200 in Rank Order

Rank	Drug	Rank	Drug
1	Valium	38	Amoxil
2	Inderal	39	Phenobarbital
3	Dyazide	40	Lopressor
4	Tylenol/Codeine	41	Naprosyn
5	Lasix Oral	42	Elavil
6	Motrin	43	Aldoril
7	Lanoxin	44	Librium
8	Ampicillin	45	Drixoral
9	Tagamet	46	Fiorinal
10	Tetracycline syst.	47	Thyroid
11	Penicillin VK	48	Ativan
12	Dalmane	49	Antivert
13	Dimetapp	50	Mycolog
14	Aldomet	51	Lomotil
15	Keflex	52	Ortho-Novum 1/50–21
16	Amoxicillin	53	Mellaril
17	Hydrochlorothiazide	54	Zomax
18	Actifed	55	Digoxin
19	E.E.S.	56	Zyloprim
20	Darvocet-N-100	57	E-Mycin
21	Erythromycin syst.	58	Ovral
22	HydroDiuril	59	Nitroglycerin
23	Slow-K	60	Timoptic
24	Premarin Oral	61	Aldactazide
25	Indocin	62	Persantine
26	Isordil	63	Lo/Ovral
27	Hygroton	64	Librax
28	V-Cillin K	65	Monistat-7
29	Empirin/Codeine	66	Atarax
30	Synthroid	67	Bactrim DS
31	Clinoril	68	Vibramycin
32	Donnatal	69	Minipress
33	Prednisone Oral	70	Naldecon
34	Dilantin Sodium	71	Ser-Ap-Es
35	Diabinese	72	Ornade
36	Benadryl Caps/Tabs	73	Percodan
37	Tranxene	74	Triavil

75	Phenergan Expect./ Codeine	115	Tenuate
76	Theo-Dur	116	Actifed-C Expectorant
77	Nitro-Bid	117	Achromycin-V
78	Insulin NPH	118	Lotrimin
79	Sinequan	119	Hydropres
80	Ceclor	120	Esidrix
81	Butazolidin Alka	121	Neosporin Ophth.
82	Nalfon	122	Septra
83	Septra DS	123	Bactrim
84	Pen-Vee-K	124	Pavabid
85	Darvon Compound-65	125	Fiorinol/Codeine
86	Apresoline	126	Poly-Vi-Flor Chewable
87	Valisone	127	Sorbitrate
88	Cortisporin Otic	128	Compazine
89	Meprobamate	129	Demulen-21
90	Potassium chloride	130	Kenalog Derm.
91	Synalgos-DC	131	Combid
92	Macrodantin	132	Lidex
93	Parafon Forte	133	Kwell
94	Diuril Oral	134	Phenergan Expectorant
95	Coumadin Oral	135	Sumycin
96	Tolinase	136	Ortho-Novum 1/50–28
97	Orinase	137	Pyridium
98	Ilosone	138	Larotid
99	Haldol	139	Nitrostat
100	Serax	140	Lo/Ovral 28
101	Enduron	141	Aldactone
102	Bentyl	142	Equagesic
103	Flagyl Oral	143	Limbitrol
104	Benadryl Elixir	144	Minocin
105	Quinidine sulfate	145	K-Lyte
106	Catapres	146	Periactin
107	Brethine	147	Butisol Sodium
108	Thorazine	148	Ovulen 21
109	Flexeril	149	Meclomen
110	Tuss-Ornade	150	Tofranil
111	Phenergan VC Expect./ Cod.	151	Stelazine
		152	Zaroxolyn
112	Phenaphen/Codeine	153	Hydrocortisone Derm.
113	Corgard	154	Bendectin
114	Talwin Tabs	155	Medrol Oral
		156	Gyne-Lotrimin

Preface

This second edition of *Top 200* has been thoroughly revised and up-dated. Twelve additional drugs appeared among the list of the top 200 during 1981, and profiles of these are contained in this edition. Information regarding the twelve that were dropped from the list may be found in the first edition of this series.

Besides the addition of these preparations, much new information is included on many of the others, especially as regards available preparations and strengths, dosage, indications for use, and precautions. Interestingly, even some older "tried and true" drugs have undergone considerable revision since the preparation of the first edition. These changes relate to more precise statements of indication, dose, precautions and even composition, thus underscoring the dynamic nature of this field and the importance of keeping abreast of the changing climate of safe drug use. More literature references are given in this edition, and it is hoped that the reader needing detailed information will consult these in order to become thoroughly familiar with the facts.

I am indebted to all those pharmaceutical manufacturers who provided me so much recent information about their respective products, and I wish here to thank them for their cooperation. I would also like to thank my daughter Karen for her typing and Dr. Robert Raffa for his help with proof-reading this edition.

R.J.T.

Preface to First Edition

This small volume contains concise summaries of the pharmacology and therapeutic uses of the 200 drugs most frequently prescribed in retail pharmacies, based on the annual National Prescription Audit. It is a handy and useful source book for medical students and residents, practicing physicians, dentists, nurses, pharmacists, teachers of pharmacology, and other health professionals who need up-to-date information on specific drugs. An opening statement on mechanism or classification, followed by indications, preparations, dosages, contraindications, adverse reactions and drug interactions, and literature references, is given for each drug. Its rank among the top 200 drugs for three years is also given.

The medical student and resident will find *Top 200* especially useful since medical school courses in pharmacology are broadly based, usually emphasizing principles and discussing drugs in groups based on chemical structure or therapeutic use. These courses do not have the time to devote to facts on the specific drugs most used in actual practice, and therefore, the new doctor or clinical clerk often lacks specific drug information when making the transition from basic science to clinical practice. *Top 200* provides this information, for it connects pharmacologic principles and information on drug groups with facts of clinical importance about the particular drugs that have the widest use. The classification in the beginning of the book serves as a guide in selecting the most appropriate drug or drugs; then reading the description provides the most pertinent clinical facts and other sources of information.

The book is organized around the actual drugs used in practice. Most are brand-name drugs. Generics are included only if they appear on the list of the most prescribed. My reasons for organizing the book in this way are several. First, these are the top 200. Second, most textbooks of pharmacology are organized so that it is not easy to get specific facts (e.g., preparations) about individual products. Finally, this selection represented a way to keep the number of drugs discussed to a manageable and practical level. In no sense, therefore, does the inclusion of any particular drug represent an endorsement by the author or publisher, nor does it mean that is necessarily the best drug in its class. Ranks for three years are given in order that the reader have some idea of the total exposure that the drug has had; also, the rank itself appears to interest many people. If no rank appears next to a year, the drug was not among the top 200 that year.

In order to keep the book small (and thus handy) I had to be brief in writing the individual monographs. The information is sufficient to give the reader the overview of the spectrum of actions and uses of the agent. Because the descriptions are brief I have included literature references. These, along with comprehensive textbooks of medicine and pharmacology, should be consulted for details since in no sense can a small volume such as this convey all the information needed by the practitioner.

In most cases quantitative information is included in the sections on adverse reactions since it is the author's conviction that this kind of information is more useful in the assessment of drug risk than a mere listing of untoward effects that have occurred. For this information I have drawn heavily from the published data of the Boston Collaborative Drug Surveillance Program.

Pharmacology is a dynamic field. New drugs are continually appearing and new uses for and new information about existing drugs accmulate rapidly. The information contained here represents that known to me at the time this book went to press. Every attempt was made to use only the most reliable sources and to edit the information carefully. Yet even as you read this, the body of information is growing and the pattern of drug usage is changing. I plan to up-date this book annually in order to provide the latest and most pertinent facts about the most prescribed drugs. I hope this series of volumes will be useful to both practitioners and teachers and will help provide improved care to the millions of patients who depend on us.

I would like to thank all the people who helped me in writing this book, but that would be difficult since the authors of every published paper that I read would have to be mentioned, even those whose works I didn't cite. Thus, I'll just thank those who helped directly: My friends at Temple University School of Medicine, J. Cavallaro, R. Incollingo, P. McGonigle, R. Murray, F. Porreca, R. Raffa, and M. J. Robinson, who helped gather the information; Margaret Staub, my daughters Diane and Karen, and my wife Theresa, who typed (several times because of revisions) the manuscript. The very capable professionals at Springer-Verlag; Berta Steiner, Production Supervisor; Chet Van Wert, Associate Medical Editor; Gabriele Schmidt, Editorial Assistant; Susan Bair, Sales Manager; and especially Larry Carter, Medical Editor, who guided this work from its inception.

R.J.T.
Philadelphia, 1981

ACHROMYCIN®-V (Lederle)
Tetracycline HCl

1981:117
1980: 93
1979: 75

Tetracyclines are mainly bacteriostatic and are thought to exert their antimicrobial effect by the inhibition of protein synthesis in a wide range of gram-negative and gram-positive organisms. Tetracyclines are readily absorbed and bind to plasma proteins.

INDICATIONS

Tetracyclines are indicated in infections caused by the following: Rickettsiae, *Mycoplasma pneumonia*, agents of psittacosis and ornithosis, agents of lymphogranuloma venereum and granuloma inguinale, and the spirochetal agent of relapsing fever (*Borrelia recurrentis*). The following gram-negative microorganisms are also sensitive: *Haemophilus ducreyi*, *Pasteurella* species, *Bartonella bacilliformis*, *Bacteroides* species, *Vibrio comma* and *Vibrio fetus* and *Brucella* species (in conjunction with streptomycin). *Tetracyclines* are alternates to penicillin in treating infections due to: *Neisseria gonorrhea*, *Treponema pallidum* and *Treponema pertenue*, *Listeria*, *Clostridium*, *Bacillus anthracis*, *Fusobacterium fusiforme* (Vincent's infection) and *Actinomyces* species. Certain other gram-positive and gram-negative microorganisms may be treated with tetracyclines when bacteriologic testing indicates appropriate susceptibility. *Tetracyclines are* usually not useful in streptococcal diseases; they have been successfully used in the management of acne. Other indications are in the treatment of trachoma and in inclusion conjunctivitis.

PREPARATIONS

Capsules: 250 and 500 mg. Oral suspension: 125 mg/5 ml. Also available for intra-

1

muscular use in vials containing 100 or 250 mg tetracycline HCl and for intravenous use in vials containing 250 or 500 mg tetracycline HCl.

DOSAGE

Oral. Adults: 250–500 mg every 6 hours. Children over 8 years: 25–50 mg/kg body weight daily in four divided doses. *Intravenous.* Adults: 250–500 mg twice daily at 12 hour intervals. Children over 8 years: 10–20 mg/kg body weight daily in divided doses every 8–12 hours. *Intramuscular.* Adults: 250 mg once daily or 300 mg daily in divided doses at 8–12 hour-intervals. Children (8 years or older): 15–25 mg/kg daily up to 250 mg per single daily injection. Dosage may be divided and given at 8–12 hour-intervals. (This route may be painful; injection should be deep into a large muscle mass; oral therapy is preferred.)

When treating syphilis, a total of 30–40 g in equally divided doses over a period of 10–15 days should be given orally. Gonorrhea patients sensitive to penicillin may be treated with tetracycline administered as an oral dose of 1–5 g followed by 0.5 g every 6 hours for 4 days to a total of 9 g. Therapy should continue for 24–48 hours after signs and symptoms disappear. Streptococcal infections that are responsive should be treated for at least 10 days.

CONTRAINDICATIONS AND PRECAUTIONS

Known hypersensitivity to any tetracycline is a contraindication. Caution must be exercised in patients with renal or hepatic problems. The use of tetracyclines during the last half of pregnancy (tooth development phase) may lead to permanent discoloration of the teeth of the offspring. Infants and children under 8 years who

2

use these drugs can experience tooth discoloration.

Gastrointestinal disturbances (nausea and vomiting) are the most common adverse effects; tooth discoloration (as described above) can occur. Less frequent adverse reactions include malabsorption, enterocolitis, photosensitivity and various sensitivity reactions. Superinfection, rise in BUN and renal damage may occur. Other reactions occur, but are rare. Among 1172 patients on tetracyclines studied in the Boston Collaborative Drug Surveillance Program 73 patients had adverse reactions as follows: gastrointestinal disturbances (41), superinfection (9), rise in BUN (8), sensitivity reactions (8), injection site complications (5), and "other" (2). These drugs interact with oral antacids, bismuth subsalicylate, oral contraceptives, oral iron, methoxyflurane, and zinc sulfate. Because tetracyclines may depress plasma prothrombin activity, patients on anticoagulant therapy may require lower doses of the anticoagulant.

LITERATURE

Am Acad Dermatol (Ad Hoc Committee on Antibiotics): Arch Dermatol 111:1630, 1975; Finland, M. Clin Pharmacol Ther 15:3, 1974 (commentary on tetracyclines); Johnson, AH: Semin Drug Treat 2:331, 1972 (adverse effects); Medical Letter 24:21, 1982 (choice of antimicrobial); Siegel, D: NY State J Med 78:950 and 1115, 1978 (reviews on tetracyclines).

ACTIFED® (Burroughs Wellcome)
Triprolidine HCl
Pseudoephedrine HCl

1981:18
1980:14
1979:11

Actifed is an antihistamine and decongestant. Its actions are due to those of its constituents. Triprolidine HCl is a potent antihistamine. Pseudoephedrine is a naturally occurring dextrostereoisomer of ephedrine and is classified as a sympathomimetic amine. The action of pseudoephedrine is apparently more specific on the blood vessels of the nasal and respiratory tract mucous membranes and less specific for the blood vessels of the systemic circulation. Actifed tablets and syrup appear to provide symptomatic relief by the rapid and sustained decongestant effect of pseudoephedrine together with the antihistaminic action of triprolidine.

INDICATIONS	Actifed is effective for the symptomatic treatment of seasonal and perennial allergic rhinitis.
PREPARATIONS	Tablets: triprolidine HCl 2.5 mg and pseudoephedrine HCl 60 mg. Syrup: 5 ml contains triprolidine HCl 1.25 mg and pseudoephedrine HCl 30 mg.
DOSAGE	Adults: 1 tablet three to four times daily or 10 ml (2 teaspoons) three to four times daily. Children, 6–12 years: half of the adult dosage; 4–6 years; ¾ teaspoon of syrup three to four times daily; 2–4 years: ½ teaspoon of syrup three to four times daily; 4 months to 2 years: ¼ teaspoon of syrup three to four times daily.
CONTRAINDICATIONS AND PRECAUTIONS	Not for use in the treatment of lower respiratory symptoms including asthma; not for newborn or premature infants; not for nursing mothers; not for individuals with hypersensitivity to the constituents or in those on monoamine oxidase inhibitors.

ADVERSE REACTIONS	Most frequently seen are sedation, sleepiness, dizziness, dryness of mouth, nose and throat. Also reported: effects on the cardiovascular system on the hematologic system as well as urticaria, photosensitivity, nervous system disturbances and difficulty in urination.
LITERATURE	Diamond, L, et al: Ann Allergy 47:87, 1981; Empey, DW, et al: Ann Allergy 34:41, 1975; Britton, MG, et al: Br J Clin Pharmacol 6:51, 1978; Irwin, RS, et al: Cough. Comprehensive review. Arch Intern Med 137:1186, 1977.

ACTIFED-C® Expectorant (Burroughs Wellcome)
Triprolidine HCl
Pseudoephedrine HCl
Codeine phosphate
Guaifenesin

1981:116
1980:105
1979:110

Actifed-C Expectorant is used in both wet and dry coughs and is effective in both infectious and allergic conditions. It may be particularly useful in the coughing, wheezing stage of respiratory allergies. Guaifenesin reduces the viscosity of the secretions, thereby increasing the efficiency of the cough reflex and the ciliary action in removing accumulated secretions from the trachea and bronchi. Codeine is an effective cough suppressant. (See ACTIFED).

INDICATIONS	Actifed-C Expectorant is indicated for the relief of cough and conditions such as the common cold, acute bronchitis, allergic asthma, bronchiolitis, croup, emphysema, and tracheobronchitis.
PREPARATIONS	One pint and one gallon bottles. Each teaspoon (5 ml) contains codeine phosphate

5

10 mg, triprolidine HCl 2 mg, pseu-doephedrine HCl 30 mg, guaifenesin 100 mg, with methylparaben 0.1% and sodium benzoate 0.1% preservatives.

DOSAGE

Four times daily as follows. Adults: 2 tea-spoons. Children 7 to 12 years: 1 tea-spoon; 2 to 6 years: ½ teaspoon.

CONTRAINDICATIONS
AND PRECAUTIONS

Not for use in patients with hypertension; used with caution in pregnant women since information on safety during preg-nancy is not adequate. (See ACTIFED).

ADVERSE REACTIONS

See ACTIFED; codeine may be habit forming.

LITERATURE

Empey, DW, et al: Ann Allergy 34:41, 1975; Britton, MG, et al: Br J Clin Pharma-col 6:51, 1978; Irwin, RS, et al: Cough. Comprehensive review. Arch Intern Med 137:1186, 1977.

ALDACTAZIDE® (Searle)
Spironolactone
Hydrochlorothiazide

1981:61
1980:54
1979:58

The diuretic effect of spironolactone is due to its action as an aldo-sterone antagonist. Hydrochlorothiazide promotes the excretion of sodium and water mainly by inhibiting their reabsorption in the cortical diluting segment of the renal tubule. Aldactazide lowers systolic and diastolic blood pressure in many patients with hyperten-sion even when aldosterone secretion is within normal limits.

INDICATIONS

To relieve edematous conditions in pa-tients with congestive heart failure when the patient is only partially responsive to or intolerant of other therapeutic mea-sures. In patients with cirrhosis of the liver accompanied by edema and/or ascites; for patients with nephrotic syndrome, and those with essential hypertension in whom other treatments are considered inappropriate.

PREPARATIONS

Tablets: 25 mg spironolactone and 25 mg hydrochlorothiazide and in tablets containing 50 mg of each ingredient.

DOSAGE

The usual adult dosage for treating essential hypertension is 2–4 tablets/day. For edema in adults the usual maintenance dose is 1 tablet four times daily. For treating edema in children the usual daily dosage is that which delivers 0.75–1.5 mg spironolactone/lb body weight (1.65–3.3 mg/kg).

CONTRAINDICATIONS AND PRECAUTIONS

Aldactazide is contraindicated in patients with anuria, impaired renal function or hyperkalemia. It is also contraindicated in patients allergic to thiazide diuretics or to other sulfonamide-derived drugs. It may also be contraindicated in cases of acute or severe hepatic failure.

ADVERSE REACTIONS

The highest incidence of adverse reactions to Aldactazide among 361 patients studied in the Boston Collaborative Drug Surveillance Program (BCDSP) was dehydration, which occurred in 21 patients. Other reactions found by BCDSP were hyperkalemia (6), hypokalemia (6), elevation of uric acid (4), gastrointestinal disturbances (4), hyponatremia (3), and CNS disturbances (1). It is noteworthy that fixed-dose combination drugs such as Aldactazide are not recommended for initial therapy of edema or hypertension. The unwanted effects of this preparation are those of its individual ingredients. (See ALDACTONE and HYDROCHLOROTHIAZIDE for further information on

adverse reactions and possible drug interactions)

LITERATURE   Medical Letter 23:45, 1981; Seller, RH.
                    et al: Arch Intern Med 113:350, 1964;
                    Winer, BM, et al: JAMA 204:775, 1968.

ALDACTONE® (Searle)   1981:141
Spironolactone   1980:144
                                             1979:147

Aldactone (spironolactone) is a pharmacologic antagonist of aldo-
sterone. It causes increased excretion of sodium and water while
potassium is retained.

INDICATIONS   Indicated in the management of primary
                    hyperaldosteronism where it is useful in
                    diagnosis, in short-term preoperative
                    treatment, as maintenance in nonsurgical
                    cases involving aldosterone-producing
                    adenomas, and as maintenance in idio-
                    pathic hyperaldosteronism. It is used in
                    edema associated with the following: con-
                    gestive heart failure in patients who do
                    not respond well to other therapeutic
                    measures, cirrhosis of the liver accompa-
                    nied by edema and/or ascites, and the ne-
                    phrotic patient. In essential hypertension,
                    aldactone is indicated for patients who
                    cannot be adequately treated with other
                    agents. It is used in patients with hypo-
                    kalemia, and is indicated for the prophy-
                    laxis of hypokalemia in digitalized pa-
                    tients.

PREPARATIONS   Tablets: 25 mg or 100 mg spironolactone.

DOSAGE   For treating edema in adults an initial
                    daily dosage of 100 mg administered in

single or divided doses is recommended but may range from 25 to 200 mg/day. For treating edema in children the dosage is based on body weight: 1.5 mg/lb of body weight daily. For treating essential hypertension the daily adult dose is 50–100 mg. For treating hypokalemia the adult daily dosage is 25–100 mg.

CONTRAINDICATIONS AND PRECAUTIONS

Aldactone is contraindicated in patients with anuria, acute renal insufficiency, impaired renal function, or hyperkalemia.

ADVERSE REACTIONS

Of 788 patients on Aldactone studied by the Boston Collaborative Drug Surveillance Program (BCDSP) the highest incidence of unwanted effects was for hyperkalemia (68 patients). BCDSP also found dehydration (27), hyponatremia (19), gastrointestinal disturbances (18), neurologic disturbances (16), rash (4), gynecomastia (2), and "other" (10). The study found sixteen adverse reactions considered to be life threatening. Death was attributed in part to spironolactone in three cases. Also reported are irregular menses, postmenopausal bleeding. Carcinoma of the breast has been reported, but a cause-effect relation has not been established. Incidences of impotency in men have been reported. It should be noted that spironolactone can enhance the actions of digoxin and, in association with potassium salts, spironolactone can produce hyperkalemia.

LITERATURE

Adlin, VE, et al: Arch Intern Med 130:855, 1972; McMahon, FG: Management of Essential Hypertensions, Mount Kisco, New York, Futura Publishing, 1978 pp 132–150; Medical Letter 23:45, 1981; Winer, BM, et al: JAMA 204(9):775, 1968.

9

ALDOMET® (Merck Sharp & Dohme)
Methyldopa

1981:14
1980:13
1979:12

The precise mechanism whereby methyldopa lowers blood pressure is not completely known, yet its antihypertensive effect is probably due to metabolism to alpha-methylnorepinephrine, which then lowers arterial pressure by stimulation of the central inhibitory alpha-adrenergic receptors. False neurotransmission and/or reduction of plasma renin activity may also contribute to the action.

INDICATIONS	Aldomet is used to treat hypertension.
PREPARATIONS	Tablets: 125, 250, and 500 mg.
DOSAGE	Usual daily adult dose is 500 mg to 2.0 g in two to four doses. Maximum recommended daily dose is 3.0 g. When used in combination the daily dosage should be 500 mg in divided doses. In children the initial dosage is based on 10 mg/kg body weight daily in two to four doses and may be adjusted to achieve an adequate response.
CONTRAINDICATIONS AND PRECAUTIONS	Active hepatic disease or if previous methyldopa therapy has been associated with liver disorders.
ADVERSE REACTIONS	Orthostatic hypotension; CNS depression (drowsiness, vertigo, dysarthria); rise in BUN; gastrointestinal disturbances. Hematologic abnormalities, including Coombs positivity, and occasionally hemolytic anemia may appear. Hepatic damage has been reported but did not occur in a series of 647 patients studied in the Boston Collaborative Drug Surveillance Program. Increased haloperidol and lithium toxicity may occur with methyldopa.

LITERATURE

Medical Letter 23:45, 1981; Page LB, Sidd, JJ: N Engl J Med 287:960–967, 1018–1023, 1074–1081, 1972 (several articles on the management of primary hypertension); Breckenridge, A, et al: Lancet 1:533, 1968; Beanlands, DS, et al: Clin Invest Med 1:139, 1978; Oberman, A, et al: Clin Ther 2:134, 1979; Walker, BR, et al: Clin Pharmacol Ther 25:252, 1979.

ALDORIL® (Merck Sharp & Dohme)
Methyldopa
Hydrochlorothiazide

1981:43
1980:42
1979:39

Methyldopa is an antihypertensive whose mechanism has not been conclusively demonstrated but is probably due to the effect on metabolism to alpha-methylnorepinephrine which then lowers arterial pressure by stimulation of central inhibitory alpha-adrenergic receptors. Hydrochlorothiazide is a diuretic and antihypertensive; it affects the renal tubular mechanism of electrolyte reabsorption.

INDICATIONS	Hypertension
PREPARATIONS	Tablets numbered ALDORIL-15, 25, 30, and 50 with compositions of (methyldopa, hydrochlorothiazide) as follows: #15 (250 mg, 15 mg), #25 (250 mg, 25 mg), #30 (500 mg, 30 mg), and #50 (500 mg, 50 mg)
DOSAGE	This is a fixed combination drug and is not indicated for initial therapy of hypertension. Therapy should be titrated to the individual patient. The usual dosage is 1 tablet of either #15, #25, #30, #50, two or three times a day in the first 48 hours. The daily dosage should then be

11

adjusted at intervals of not less than 2 days, until an adequate response is achieved. The maximum recommended daily dosage is 3.0 g of methyldopa and 100 to 200 mg of hydrochlorothiazide.

CONTRAINDICATIONS AND PRECAUTIONS

Active hepatic disease or if previous methyldopa therapy has been associated with liver disorders. Anuria is a contraindication as is sensitivity to methyldopa or to hydrochlorothiazide or other sulfonamide-derived drugs.

ADVERSE REACTIONS

The adverse reactions are those associated with the constituents. (See ALDOMET and HYDROCHLOROTHIAZIDE)

LITERATURE

Hollifield, JW, Moore, L: Clin Ther 2(Suppl A):38, 1979; Agodoa, L: Clin Ther 2(Suppl A): 44, 1979; Hollifield, JW, Slaton, PE, Jr: Curr Ther Res Clin Exp 24:818, 1978; Medical Letter 23:45, 1981.

AMBENYL® EXPECTORANT (Marion)

1981:191
1980:161
1979:169

Codeine
Bromodiphenhydramine HCl
Diphenhydramine HCl
Ammonium chloride
Potassium guaiacolsulfonate
Menthol
Alcohol

Ambenyl is a combination of two antihistaminic agents along with well-recognized compounds that exhibit expectorant and antitussive properties. Diphenhydramine HCl, in addition to being a potent antihistaminic, also possesses antitussive actions.

INDICATIONS	Ambenyl is indicated as an antitussive and expectorant for control of cough due to cold or allergy.
PREPARATIONS	Each 5 ml contains codeine sulfate 10 mg, bromodiphenhydramine HCl 3.75 mg, diphenhydramine HCl 8.75 mg, ammonium chloride 80 mg, potassium guaiacolsulfonate 80 mg, menthol 0.5 mg, and alcohol 5%.
DOSAGE	Adults: 1 or 2 teaspoons every 4–6 hours, not to exceed 12 teaspoons in 24 hours. Children, 6 to 12 years of age: ½–1 teaspoon every 6 hours; 2–6 years of age: ¼–½ teaspoon every 6 hours. (The total intake of codeine sulfate in children should not exceed 1 mg/kg body weight/day.) Not recommended for children under 2 years of age.
CONTRAINDICATIONS AND PRECAUTIONS	This preparation is contraindicated in patients with hypersensitivity to any of the components, asthmatic attack, narrow-angle glaucoma, prostatic hypertrophy, stenosing peptic ulcer, pyloroduodenal obstruction or bladder-neck obstruction. Use with caution during pregnancy and lactation and in association with other CNS depressants such as alcohol, hypnotics, and tranquilizers.
ADVERSE REACTIONS	The following may occur: drowsiness, confusion, restlessness, nausea, diarrhea, vomiting, blurred vision, diplopia, constipation, difficulty in urination, nasal stuffiness, vertigo, palpitations, headache, insomnia, urticaria, drug rash, tightness of the chest and wheezing, dryness of mouth, nose, and throat, tingling and weakness of hands, photosensitivity, hemolytic anemia, hypotension and epigastric distress.

LITERATURE   Irwin, RS, et al: Arch Intern Med 137:1186, 1977 (comprehensive review of cough).

AMINOPHYLLINE
Aminophylline

1981:186
1980:157
1979:154

Aminophylline is converted in the body to theophylline, the active agent responsible for its actions which are typical of xanthine derivatives: direct relaxation of bronchial smooth muscle and pulmonary blood vessels, coronary vasodilation, diuresis, cardiac stimulation, skeletal muscle stimulation, and cerebral stimulation. Aminophylline increases both the depth and rate of respiration, and it increases cardiac output and renal blood flow.

INDICATIONS

Bronchial asthma, status asthmaticus, congestive heart failure, Cheyne-Stokes respiration, and the reduction of coughing, expectoration and exertional dyspnea in emphysema patients, and for cardiac paroxysmal dyspnea; it is also a diuretic.

PREPARATIONS

Tablets: 100 or 200 mg of aminophylline. For parenteral use as intravenous injection in ampuls of 10 ml (250 mg) or 20 ml (500 mg) and as intramuscular injection in ampuls of 2 ml (500 mg).

DOSAGE

The oral dose for adults is adjusted to patient need and is in the range 600–1600 mg daily administered in three or four divided doses. The oral dose in children is based on body weight and is usually 12 mg/kg daily administered in four divided doses. Adjustment of the dose in children is based on the response.

When given intravenously in adults the dose is 250–500 mg *given slowly* over a period of 20 minutes or more. When congestive failure or hepatic disease is present the dose should be reduced by 25%. Intravenous dosage in children is 6 mg/kg body weight, given slowly over a period of 20 minutes or more. When the intramuscular route is used the usual dose for adults and children is 5–6 mg/kg body weight every 6–8 hours. Oral therapy should be used as soon as adequate improvement occurs.

CONTRAINDICATIONS AND PRECAUTIONS

Aminophylline is contraindicated in patients with active peptic ulcer disease or with known hypersensitivity to aminophylline or theophylline. Not for use during pregnancy under normal circumstances. Many common foods and beverages (eg, chocolate, cola beverages, coffee and tea) contain xanthines and should be taken cautiously during aminophylline treatment.

ADVERSE REACTIONS

The most common adverse reactions are gastrointestinal, central (dizziness and vertigo), cardiovascular (palpitations, tachycardia and flushing), respiratory (increased rate) and dermatologic. Many brands of erythromycin and troleandomycin will enhance the theophylline levels whereas smoking decreases its effects. The effects of lithium and propranolol may be decreased when used concurrently with aminophylline. In the Boston Collaborative Drug Surveillance Program 1819 patients taking aminophylline were observed. The highest incidence of adverse reactions included gastrointestinal disturbances (9.3%), tachycardia or palpitations (1.0%), vertigo or headache (0.04%), hypotension (0.3%) and CNS disturbances (0.2%). Other reactions were variable and of low incidence. Among this group of patients there were four serious adverse reactions attributed to aminophylline: two episodes of hypotension and two of severe vomiting or diarrhea.

LITERATURE   Mitenko, PA, Ogilvie, RI: N Engl J Med 289:600, 1973 (on intravenous dosing with theophylline); Tong, TG: Drug Intel Clin Pharm 7:156, 1973 (review article).

AMITRIPTYLINE HCl

1981:184
1980: —
1979: —

Amitriptyline is an antidepressant with antianxiety action and a sedative component. Its precise mechanism is not known; it is not a monoamine oxidase inhibitor and it does not act primarily by stimulating the central nervous system. Amitriptyline is known to inhibit the membrane mechanism responsible for reuptake of norepinephrine into adrenergic neurons.

INDICATIONS   Amitriptyline HCl is used for the relief of symptoms of depression. Endogenous depression is more likely to be alleviated than are other depressive states.

PREPARATIONS   Tablets 10, 25, 50, 75, 100, and 150 mg. Sterile solution for intramuscular injection. Each ml of the solution contains amitriptyline HCl 10 mg, dextrose 44 mg, water for injection, and preservatives.

DOSAGE   The initial daily dosage for adults is 75 mg in divided doses and may be increased to 150 mg if necessary. Alternatively therapy may be initiated with 50–100 mg at bedtime. Lower doses are recommended for adolescent and elderly patients (eg, 10 mg, three times a day, with 20 mg at bedtime.) Adequate response may take 30 days to develop. Maintenance dosage is 50–100 mg daily. When therapy is initiated with the parental route (I.M.) 20 or 30 mg daily (2–3 ml) four times a day may be used. Amitriptyline is not for patients under 12 years of age.

CONTRAINDICATIONS AND PRECAUTIONS

This drug is contraindicated in patients with known hypersensitivity. Also, it should not be used concomitantly with MAO inhibitors. (Wait 14 days between the last dose of an MAO inhibitor if Amitriptyline is being started.) Amitriptyline is contraindicated during the acute recovery phase following myocardial infarction.

ADVERSE REACTIONS

Adverse reactions include effects on the CNS (drowsiness and confusion), the cardiovascular system, the gastrointestinal system and the hematologic system as well as anticholinergic effects and allergic reactions. Among 309 patients receiving Amitriptyline and followed in the Boston Collaborative Drug Surveillance Program, 40 patients experienced side effects as follows: drowsiness (20), CNS excitation (11), anticholinergic reactions (5), headache or tinnitus (2), and cardiovascular effects consisting of arrhythmias and hypotension (2).

Amitriptyline may block the antihypertensive action of guanethidine and similarly acting drugs and may enhance the response to alcohol and the effects of barbiturates and other CNS depressants.

LITERATURE

Cecchini, S, et al, J Int Med Res 6:388, 1978; Cutler, NR, Heiser, JF: JAMA 240:2264, 1978; Kampman, R, et al: Acta Psychiatr Scand 58:142, 1978; Klerman, GL, Hirschfeld, RMA: JAMA 240:1403, 1978.

AMOXICILLIN

1981:16
1980:19
1979:35

Amoxicillin, an analogue of ampicillin, is a semisynthetic antibiotic with essentially the same broad spectrum of bacteriocidal activity as ampicillin against many gram-positive and certain gram-negative microorganisms. Like ampicillin, this drug is susceptible to destruction by penicillinase. It is stable in the presence of gastric acid ànd may be given without regard to meals. It is rapidly absorbed after oral administration.

INDICATIONS

Amoxicillin is indicated in the treatment of infections due to strains of the following organisms: gram-negative, including *H. influenzae, E. coli, P. mirabilis,* and *N. gonorrhoeae;* gram-positive organisms such as streptococci, *D. pneumoniae,* and non-penicillinaise-producing staphylococci. Amoxicillin seems less effective than ampicillin for treating shigellosis. Infections of skin, soft tissues, lower respiratory, and urinary tracts caused by susceptible strains of the above microorganisms respond well to amoxicillin.

PREPARATIONS

Capsules: 250 and 500 mg. Chewable tablets: 125 and 250 mg. Oral suspension and powder for suspension: 125 and 250 mg/ml. (See also AMOXIL and LARO-TID)

DOSAGE

The usual oral dosage range in adults and *children weighing more than 20 kg* is 250–500 mg every 8 hours. For children less than 20 kg, 20–40 mg/kg daily in divided doses at 8 hour intervals. The higher doses are used in lower respiratory tract infections. For uncomplicated gonococcal infections in men and women oral amoxicillin 3 g plus 1 g of probenecid is given in a single dose, and in children *2 years or older,* 50 mg/kg amoxicillin plus 25 mg/kg of probenecid as a single dose.

CONTRAINDICATIONS
AND PRECAUTIONS

Known hypersensitivity to penicillins is a contraindication.

ADVERSE REACTIONS

Nausea, vomiting, and diarrhea (less severe than with ampicillin) can occur. Hypersensitivity reactions including rash, fever, serum sickness-like effects, anemia, eosinophilia, and other blood effects have been reported. Anaphylactic reactions occur much less frequently with oral penicillins than with parenterally administered penicillins.

LITERATURE

Brogden, RN, et al: Drugs 9:88, 1975 (review on amoxicillin); Eichenwald, HF, McCracken, GH, Jr: J Pediatr 93:337, 1978 (review of antimicrobials); Medical Letter 24:21, 1982 (choice of antimicrobial); Medical Letter 23:69, 1981 (urinary tract infections); Neu, HC: Drugs 9:81, 1975 (editorial on new broad-spectrum penicillin). For treatment of gonorrhea in young children, see recommendation by Center for Disease Control: Ann Intern Med 90:809, 1979.

AMOXIL® (Beecham)
Amoxicillin trihydrate

1981:38
1980:48
1979:64

Amoxicillin, an analogue of ampicillin, is a semisynthetic antibiotic with essentially the same broad spectrum of bacteriocidal activity as ampicillin against many gram-positive and certain gram-negative microorganisms. Like ampicillin, this drug is susceptible to destruction by penicillinase. It is stable in the presence of gastric acid and may be given without regard to meals. It is rapidly absorbed after oral administration.

INDICATIONS

Amoxicillin is indicated in the treatment of infections due to strains of the following organisms: gram-negative, including *H. influenzae, E. coli, P. mirabilis* and *N. gonorrhoeae;* gram-positive organisms such as streptococci, *D. pneumoniae,* and non-penicillinase-producing staphylococci. Amoxicillin seems less effective than ampicillin for treating shigellosis. Infections of skin, soft tissues, lower respiratory, and urinary tracts caused by susceptible strains of the above microorganisms respond well to amoxicillin.

PREPARATIONS

Capsules: 250 and 500 mg. Chewable tablets: 125 and 250 mg. Oral suspension: 125 mg/5 ml and 250 mg/5 ml after reconstitution. Pediatric drops: each 1 ml of the reconstituted suspension contains 50 mg.

DOSAGE

The usual oral dosage range in adults and *children weighing more than 20 kg* is 250–500 mg every 8 hours. For children less than 20 kg, 20–40 mg/kg daily in divided doses at 8 hour intervals. The higher doses are used in lower respiratory tract infections. For uncomplicated gonococcal infections in men and women oral amoxicillin 3 g plus 1 g of probenecid is given in a single dose, and in children *2 years or older,* 50 mg/kg amoxicillin plus 25 mg/kg of probenecid as a single dose.

CONTRAINDICATIONS AND PRECAUTIONS

Known hypersensitivity to penicillins is a contraindication.

ADVERSE REACTIONS

Nausea, vomiting, and diarrhea (less severe than with ampicillin) can occur. Hy-

20

persensitivity reactions including rash, fever, serum sickness-like effects, anemia, eosinophilia, and other blood effects have been reported. Anaphylactic reactions occur much less frequently with oral penicillins than with parenterally administered penicillins.

LITERATURE

Brogden, RN, et al: Drugs 9:88, 1975 (review on amoxicillin); Eichenwald, HF, McCracken, GH, Jr: J Pediatr 93:337, 1978 (review of antimicrobials); Medical Letter 24:21, 1982 (choice of antimicrobials); Medical Letter 23:69, 1981 (urinary tract infections), Neu, HC: Drugs 9:81, 1975 (editorial on new broad-spectrum penicillin). For treatment of gonorrhea in young children, see recommendation by Center for Disease Control; Ann Intern Med 90:809, 1979.

AMPICILLIN

1981:8
1980:6
1979:3

Ampicillin is a semisynthetic penicillin derived from the basic penicillin nucleus and has a broader spectrum than penicillin G or V. It is effective against many gram-positive and certain gram-negative microorganisms, such as *H. influenzae, E. coli,* and *Proteus mirabilis.* Ampicillin is stable in acid and is well absorbed after oral administration. The administration of probenecid leads to increased plasma concentrations of ampicillin. Mircrobial resistance to ampicillin is increasing. Many strains of *E. coli, P. mirabilis,* and *Salmonella* are now resistant to ampicillin. Most strains of *Shigella* and *Enterobacter* are presently insensitive.

INDICATIONS

For treatment of infections caused by susceptible strains of *E. coli, H. influenzae, P.*

21

mirabilis, N. gonorrhoeae, Shigella, Salmonella and enterococci. Ampicillin is also indicated in certain infections caused by susceptible gram-positive organisms, such as penicillin G-sensitive staphylococci, streptococci, and pneumococci. The primary clinical indications for ampicillin are urinary, respiratory and gastrointestinal tract infections and bacterial otitis and meningitis in children. Ampicillin is used in treating gonorrhea (althugh penicillin G is preferred) and is used to treat typhoid fever resistant to chloramphenicol.

PREPARATIONS

Capsules: 250 and 500 mg. Powder for suspension: 125, 250, and 500 mg/5 ml. Suspension: 125 and 250 mg/5 ml. Tablets: 125 mg.

DOSAGE

The usual *oral* dosage range in adults and children weighing more than 20 kg is 250–500 mg four times daily; for children less than 20 kg the range is 50–100 mg/kg body weight daily, given in divided doses at 6 hour intervals. The *intramuscular* and *intravenous* dosage range is as follows: adults and children over 20 kg: 200–500 mg four times daily at 6 hour intervals; children less than 20 kg: 25–100 mg/kg body weight daily in divided doses every 6 hours (but not to exceed adult dose). For bacterial meningitis much higher doses are used (see package insert). For gonorrhea, 1 g probenecid plus 3.5 g ampicillin is given orally as a single dose. (For infants less than 7 days, see the package insert.)

CONTRAINDICATIONS AND PRECAUTIONS

Patients with a history of hypersensitivity to the penicillins. Safe use in pregnancy has not been established.

ADVERSE REACTIONS

Rashes and gastrointestinal disturbances (mainly diarrhea) are the most common adverse effects. Among 2344 patients on ampicillin in the Boston Collaborative Drug Surveillance Program 249 patients had adverse effects as follows: rash or pruritis (116), gastrointestinal disturbances (95), injection site complications (9), superinfection (15), drug fever (7), and "other" (7).

LITERATURE

Caldwell, JR, Cluff, LE, JAMA 230:77, 1974 (adverse reactions to antimicrobials); Ehrnebo, M, et al: J Pharmacokinet Biopharm 7:429, 1979 (pharmacokinetics of ampicillin); Eichenwald, HF, and McCracken, GH, Jr: J Pediatr 93:337, 1978; Mandell, GL, Sande, MA: In The Pharmacological Basis of Therapeutics, 6th ed (Gilman, AG, Goodman, LS, Gilman, A, eds). New York, Macmillan, 1980, Chapter 50; Medical Letter 24:21, 1982 (choice of antimicrobials).

ANTIVERT® (Roerig)
Meclizine HCl

1981:49
1980:44
1979:47

Antivert is an antihistamine and antinausea agent.

INDICATIONS

Antivert is effective in the management of the nausea, vomiting, and dizziness associated with motion sickness. It is possibly effective in the management of vertigo associated with diseases affecting the vestibular system.

PREPARATIONS

Tablets: 12.5 and 25 mg.

DOSAGE

For motion sickness prevention the initial dose is 25–50 mg taken 1 hour before the

23

journey. Thereafter the dose may be repeated every 24 hours for the duration of the journey. For control of vertigo associated with vestibular disorders the recommended dose is 25–100 mg daily, in divided dosage at intervals that depend on the degree of clinical response.

CONTRAINDICATIONS AND PRECAUTIONS

This drug is contraindicated in patients with previous hypersensitivity. This medication, or any other medication, should be used during pregnancy only if clearly necessary.

ADVERSE REACTIONS

Drowsiness and dry mouth may occur. Blurred vision has been reported but is rare.

LITERATURE

Turner, JS, Jr: South Med J 68:241, 1975; Wood, CD: Drugs 17:471, 1979.

ANUSOL-HC® (Parke-Davis)
Hydrocortisone acetate
Bismuth subgallate
Bismuth resorcin compound
Benzyl benzoate
Peruvian balsam
Zinc oxide

1981:164
1980:169
1979:183

Anusol-HC suppositories and cream help to relieve the pain, itching, and discomfort arising from irritated anorectal tissues. These preparations have a soothing lubricant action on mucous membranes and the anti-inflammatory action of hydrocortisone acetate helps reduce hyperemia and swelling. The hydrocortisone acetate is primarily effective because of its anti-inflammatory, antipruritic, and vasoconstrictive actions.

INDICATIONS	Suppositories and cream are adjunctive therapy for the symptomatic relief of the pain and discomfort in external and internal hemorrhoids, proctitis, papillitis, cryptitis, anal fissures, incomplete fistulas, and relief of local pain and discomfort following anorectal surgery. It is also indicated for the relief of pruritis ani. Anusol-HC is especially indicated when inflammation is present. After acute symptoms subside, most patients can be maintained on regular Anusol.
PREPARATIONS	Suppositories and cream.
DOSAGE	Suppositories are inserted into the anus, one in the morning and one at bedtime for 3–6 days or until the inflammation subsides. Anusol-HC cream is applied three to four times a day, after gentle bathing and drying of the anal area, for 3–6 days or until the inflammation subsides.
CONTRAINDICATIONS AND PRECAUTIONS	These preparations are contraindicated in patients with a history of hypersensitivity to any of the components of the preparation.
ADVERSE REACTIONS	The safe use of topical steroids during pregnancy has not been fully established and, therefore, these preparations should be used cautiously in pregnant women. The same precautions should be applied in children and infants. In all cases, discontinue use if irritation develops.
LITERATURE	AMA Drug Evaluations, 4th ed. AMA and Wiley, New York, 1980, pp 1006–1007. Lieberman, W: Am J Proctol 17:371, 1966; Medical Letter 10:105, 1968.

25

APRESOLINE® (Ciba)
Hydralazine HCl

1981: 86
1980: 85
1979:103

Apresoline lowers blood pressure by means of a direct relaxing action on vascular smooth muscle.

INDICATIONS	Apresoline is indicated for the treatment of essential hypertension either alone or as an adjunct to other therapy.
PREPARATIONS	Tablets: 10, 25, 50, and 100 mg. Injectable form (used only when the oral route cannot be used): 1 ml ampuls each containing 20 mg hydralazine hydrochloride and preservatives in water.
DOSAGE	When initiating therapy in adults with Apresoline as the sole therapeutic agent the dose is 10 mg four times a day for 2–4 days then followed by 25 mg four times a day for the rest of the week. For the second and subsequent weeks the dosage may be increased to 50 mg four times daily. The incidence of toxic reactions may be higher with larger doses of Apresoline. In these cases a lower dose of Apresoline may be combined with a thiazide or other antihypertensive drug. When used parenterally (only when the oral route is impossible or in emergencies) the usual dose is 20–40 mg intravenously or intramuscularly. A fall in blood pressure may occur in 10–80 minutes after injection.
CONTRAINDICATIONS AND PRECAUTIONS	Apresoline is contraindicated in patients with coronary artery disease and with mitral valvular rheumatic heart disease. It should also not be used in patients with

previous demonstration of hypersensitivity to the drug or in pregnant women.

In some patients hydralazine may produce a syndrome that resembles systemic lupus erythematosus. Common side effects include headache, palpitations, anorexia, nausea, vomiting, diarrhea, tachycardia, and angina pectoris. The Boston Collaborative Drug Surveillance Program (BCDSP) studied 223 patients on hydralazine and reported hypotension as the most frequent adverse reaction (22 patients) followed by headache (8), gastrointestinal disturbances (4), tachycardia or palpitations (3), rise in BUN (2), and "other" (2). BCDSP reported two severe adverse reactions in patients receiving parenteral hydralazine because of severe hypertension.

Less frequent adverse reactions are nasal congestion, flushing, lacrimation, conjunctivitis, peripheral neuritis, edema, dizziness, tremors, muscle cramps, and psychotic reactions. Constipation and difficulty in micturition have also been reported as have dyspnea, paralytic ileus, lymphadenopathy, splenomegaly, and blood dyscrasias. Paradoxical pressor response has also been reported.

MAO inhibitors should be used cautiously in patients receiving hydralazine. When other powerful antihypertensive drugs are used with hydralazine given parenterally the patient should be watched for any excessive fall in blood pressure.

LITERATURE   Hollander, W: Clin Ther 2(Suppl A): 11, 1979; McMahon, FG: Management of Essential Hypertension, Futura Publishing, Mount Kisko, New York, 1978, pp 209–249. *For information and references on the use of hydralazine and other vasodilators in the*

27

treatment of congestive heart failure, see Fitch-ett, DH, et al: Am J Cardiol 44(2):303, 1979; Medical Letter 20:89, 1978; Medical Letter 23:45, 1981.

ARTANE® (Lederle)
Trihexyphenidyl HCl

1981:194
1980: —
1979: —

Trihexyphenidyl HCl is a synthetic antispasmodic drug used as an adjunct in the treatment of parkinsonism. It relaxes smooth muscle, both directly and indirectly through inhibition of the parasympathetic nervous system. Its actions are similar to those of atropine, although undesirable side effects are usually less frequent and less severe than with atropine.

INDICATIONS

As an adjunct in the treatment of all forms of parkinsonism. It is also used for the control of extrapyramidal disorders caused by other CNS drugs.

PREPARATIONS

Tablets: 2 mg and 5 mg. Elixir: 2 mg/5ml. Sustained-release capsules: 5 mg.

DOSAGE

As initial therapy for parkinsonism, 1 mg (tablet or elixir form) is administered on the first day, then adjusted upward at intervals of 3 to 5 days in 2 mg increments to a total daily dosage of 6–10 mg. (Some patients, mainly postencephalitic group, may require daily doses of 12–15 mg.) When treating drug-induced parkinsonism the daily dosage range is 5 to 15 mg, although in some cases control is achieved on as little as 1 mg daily. When Artane is used with Levodopa, careful adjustment is necessary. Usually, in these cases, 3–6 mg daily of Artane is adequate. Tablets and elixir are usually tolerated best if given in 3 divided doses at mealtimes. The sustained release form is not recommended for initial therapy, but is used for convenience in maintaining control on a milligram per milligram total daily dose basis, either as a single dose after breakfast or in two divided doses 12 hours apart.

CONTRAINDICATIONS AND PRECAUTIONS

Patients to be treated with Artane should have a gonioscope evaluation and close monitoring of intraocular pressures at regular intervals. Close supervision is necessary when using Artane in patients with cardiac, liver, or kidney disorders, or with hypertension. This drug should be used cautiously in patients with glaucoma, obstructive diseases of the gastrointestinal or genitourinary tracts, in elderly patients and in elderly males with prostatic hypertrophy.

ADVERSE REACTIONS

Minor side effects, such as dryness of the mouth, blurring of vision, dizziness, mild nausea or nervousness, occur in 30 to 50% of all patients but usually become less pronounced as treatment continues. Isolated instances of supparative parotitis secondary to excessive dryness of the mouth, skin rashes, dilatation of the colon, paralytic ileus, and certain psychiatric manifestations have rarely occurred. Potential side effects are those associated with atropine-like drugs.

LITERATURE

Bianchine, JR: in *The Pharmacological Basis of Therapeutics* (Gilman, AG, Goodman, LS, Gilman, A, eds). New York, Macmillan, 1980, Chapter 21.

ATARAX® (Roerig)
Hydroxyzine HCl

1981:66
1980:66
1979:70

Atarax is broadly classified as a tranquilizer. It is not chemically related to the phenothiazines, reserpine, or meprobamate. Hydroxyzine has been shown clinically to be a true rapid-acting ataraxic; it induces calming effects in anxious, tense psychoneurotic adults and also in hyperkinetic children without apparent impairment of mental alertness. It is not a cortical depressant, but its action may be due to suppression of its activity in certain key regions in the subcortical area of the central nervous system. Experimentally, hydroxyzine has been shown to have antispasmodic properties apparently mediated through interference with the mechanism that responds to spasmogenic agents such as serotonin, acetylcholine, and histamine. It also has antihistaminic effects and a possible antiemetic effect.

INDICATIONS

Hydroxyzine is indicated for symptomatic relief of anxiety and tension associated with psychoneurosis and as an adjunct in organic disease states in which anxiety is manifested. It is also useful in the management of pruritis due to allergic conditions such as chronic urticaria and atopic and contact dermatoses, and in histamine-mediated pruritis. When used as a sedative, and after general anesthesia, hydroxyzine may potentiate meperidine and barbiturates.

PREPARATIONS

Tablets: 10, 25, 50, and 100 mg. Syrup: 10 mg per teaspoon (5 ml).

DOSAGE

For symptomatic relief of anxiety and tension, the usual adult dose is 50–100 mg four times per day. In children under 6 years the daily dose is 50 mg in divided doses; in children over 6 years the daily dose is 50–100 mg in divided doses.

In the management of pruritis the usual

adult dose is 25 mg three or four times per day whereas the dose in children is 50 mg daily in divided doses for children less than 6 years and 50–100 mg daily in divided doses for older children.

When used as a sedative for premedication and following general anesthesia the adult dose is 50–100 mg and the child's dose is 0.6 mg/kg body weight.

CONTRAINDICATIONS AND PRECAUTIONS

Hydroxyzine is contraindicated in patients with previous demonstration of hypersensitivity to the drug. Clinical data in human beings is inadequate to establish safety in early pregnancy.

ADVERSE REACTIONS

Side effects reported with recommended doses of Atarax are mild and transitory in nature. These are dry mouth, drowsiness, and involuntary motor activity. The Boston Collaborative Drug Surveillance Study found these mild side effects occurred in only 3 of 137 patients studied. Hydroxyzine may potentiate meperidine (Demerol®) and barbiturates.

LITERATURE

Baraf, CS: Curr Ther Res 19:32, 1976; Barranco, SF, Bridger, W: Curr Ther Res 22:217, 1977. Dilts, SL, et al: Am J Psychiat 134:92, 1977; Rhoades, RB, et al: J Allergy Clin Immunol 55:180, 1975; Tobias, M, et al: J Dent Child 42:453, 1975.

ATIVAN® (Wyeth)
Lorazepam

1981:48
1980:63
1979:84

Ativan, a benzodiazepine antianxiety agent, has a tranquilizing effect on the central nervous system with no appreciable effect on the respiratory or cardiovascular systems.

INDICATIONS

Ativan is indicated for the management of anxiety disorders or for the short-term relief of the symptoms of anxiety or anxiety associated with depressive symptoms. The effectiveness of Ativan in long-term use, that is, more than four months, has not been assessed by systematic clinical studies.

PREPARATIONS

Tablets: 0.5, 1.0, and 2.0 mg.

DOSAGE

The usual dosage range is 2–6 mg/day (but may vary from 1–10 mg/day) in divided doses, the largest dose being taken before bedtime. For insomnia due to anxiety, a single daily dose of 2–4 mg may be given at bedtime. For elderly or debilitated patients, an initial daily dose of 1–2 mg is recommended and should be adjusted as needed.

CONTRAINDICATIONS AND PRECAUTIONS

Lorazepam is contraindicated in patients with known sensitivity to benzodiazepines or with acute narrow angle glaucoma. Not for patients with a primary depressive disorder or psychosis.

ADVERSE REACTIONS

Adverse reactions, if they occur, are usually observed at the beginning of therapy and generally disappear on continued medication or upon decreasing the dose. In a sample of about 3,500 anxious patients, the most frequent adverse reaction to Ativan (lorazepam) is sedation (15.9%), followed by dizziness (6.9%), weakness (4.2%), and unsteadiness (3.4%). Less frequent adverse reactions are disorientation, depression, nausea, change in appetite, headache, sleep disturbance, agitation, dermatological symptoms, eye-function disturbance, together with various gastrointestinal symptoms and autonomic manifestations. The inci-

dence of sedation and unsteadiness increased with age.

LITERATURE   J Clin Psychiatry 39, No. 10, Oct, 1978
(entire issue, 10 articles). Medical Letter
23:41, 1981 (choice of benzodiazepines).

ATROMID-S® (Ayerst)
Clofibrate

1981:196
1980:138
1979: 98

Atromid-S is an antilipidemic agent for the reduction of elevated
serum lipids. It helps to lower elevated serum lipids by reducing
the very low density lipoprotein fraction rich in triglycerides. Serum
cholesterol, especially the low density lipoprotein fraction, is also
decreased, particularly in those patients whose cholesterol levels are
elevated at the outset. The mechanism of action has not been established definitively. Drug treatment should not be used for the routine
treatment of elevated blood lipids for the prevention of coronary
artery disease. Dietary therapy specific for the type of hyperlipidemia
is the initial treatment of choice and contributory diseases such as
hypothyroidism and diabetes mellitus should be looked for and adequately treated. There is not, to date, substantial evidence of a beneficial effect on cardiovascular mortality from clofibrate or any other
lipid-altering agent.

INDICATIONS   Atromid-S is indicated for Primary Dysbe-
talipoproteinemia (Type III hyperlipide-
mia) that does not respond adequately to
diet. It may be considered for the treatment of adults with very high serum tri-
glyceride levels (Types IV and V hyperlipidemia) who present risk of abdominal
pain and pancreatitis who do not respond
to dietary efforts.

PREPARATIONS   Tablets: 500 mg.

DOSAGE	The recommended initial and maintenance dose for adults is 2 g daily in divided doses. Safety and efficacy in children have not been established.
CONTRAINDICATIONS AND PRECAUTIONS	Clofibrate is contraindicated in pregnant and lactating women, in patients with hepatic and renal dysfunction, and in patients with primary biliary cirrhosis.
ADVERSE REACTIONS	Nausea, diarrhea, and other gastrointestinal disturbances can occur. Reactions reported less often than gastrointestinal ones are headache, dizziness, fatigue, muscle cramps, weakness, skin rash, urticaria and pruritis, dry hair, and alopecia. Patients with existing or suspected coronary artery disease may be at risk from drug induced arrhythmias, increased angina, claudication, and thromboembolic events. The use of clofibrate may be associated with an increased incidence of tumors and increased risk of cholelithiasis. Clofibrate enhances the effects of other acidic drugs such as phenytoin and tolbutamide. It also increases the action of oral anticoagulants, requiring in some cases about one half the usual anticoagulant dose.
LITERATURE	Coronary Drug Project. JAMA 231:360, 1975; Report of the Committee (prevention of heart disease using clofibrate). Br Heart J 40:1069, 1978.

BACTRIM® (Roche)
Trimethoprim
Sulfamethoxazole

1981:123
1980:149
1979: —

This preparation contains exactly one half the amounts of each ingredient contained in BACTRIM DS (double strength). (See BACTRIM DS)

BACTRIM® DS (Roche)
Trimethoprim
Sulfamethoxasole

1981:67
1980:76
1979:93

The combination of a folic acid antagonist and a sulfonamide inhibits two consecutive steps in the biosynthesis of nucleic acids and proteins essential to many bacteria. The two compounds are synergistic against many common urinary and other type infections.

INDICATIONS

For urinary tract infections due to susceptible strains of *E. coli, Klebsiella-Enterobacter, P. mirabilis, P. vulgaris* and *P. morganii,* shigellosis, and *Pneumocystis carinii* pneumonitis. It is also used for treating acute otitis media in children due to susceptible strains of *H. influenzae* or *S. pneumoniae* and acute exacerbations of chronic bronchitis in adults due to these microorganisms.

PREPARATIONS

Double strength tablets: 160 mg trimethoprim and 800 mg sulfamethoxazole. Tablets: 80 mg trimethoprim and 400 mg sulfamethoxazole; suspension: each teaspoon (5 ml) contains 40 mg trimethoprim and 200 mg sulfamethoxazole. Suspensions are fruit-licorice or cherry flavored for pediatric use.

For adults the usual dosage for urinary tract infections is one Bactrim DS tablet or two Bactrim tablets every 12 hours for 10–14 days. The same dosage is used for 5 days in the treatment of shigellosis. The usual dosage for children with urinary tract infections or acute otitis media is 8 mg/kg trimethoprim and 40 mg/kg sulfamethoxazole per day given in two divided doses every 12 hours for 10 days (5 days for treating shigellosis). For patients with renal impairment half the usual dose is used. For cases of severe renal impairment (creatinine clearance below 15 ml/minute) this drug is not recommended.

For treating acute exacerbations of chronic bronchitis in adults the usual dosage is one Bactrim DS tablet or two Bactrim tablets (or four teaspoons) every 12 hours for 14 days.

For treating *Pneumocystis carinii* pneumonitis the usual dose is based on patient weight: 20 mg/kg trimethoprim and 100 mg/kg sulfamethoxazole per day given in equally divided doses every 6 hours for 14 days. In children weighing 80 lb (36 kg) the dosage is 1 Bactrim DS tablet every 6 hours for 14 days. For children less than 70 lb this dosage in children may be attained by administering the following every 6 hours:

Weight		Teaspoon	Tablets
lb	kg		
18	8	1	½
35	16	2	1
53	24	3	1½
70	32	4	2

Bactrim should not be used during pregnancy or during the nursing period. Hypersensitivity to either ingredient is also a contraindication. Not for infants less than 2 months old.

ADVERSE REACTIONS

Gastrointestinal disturbances, allergic reactions, and blood dyscrasias can occur. Central nervous system reactions including muscle weakness have been reported, as have drug fever, chills, and toxic nephrosis with oliguria and anuria. Periarteritis nodosa and lupus-like phenomena have occurred. Sulfonamides can increase the anticoagulant effect of warfarin and can also enhance the action of oral hypoglycemics.

LITERATURE

Finland, M, Kass, EH (eds): J Infect Dis 128(Suppl):425, 1972 (see also Drugs 1:7, 1971); Kunin, CM, et al: JAMA 239:2588, 1978; Lau, WK, Young, LS: N Engl J Med 295:716, 1976; Medical Letter 23:69, 1981; 23:102, 1981.

BENADRYL® CAPSULES/TABLETS (Parke-Davis)
Diphenhydramine HCl

1981:36
1980:33
1979:29

Benadryl is an antihistamine. It has anticholinergic or drying actions, a central antitussive effect, an antiemetic effect and sedative side effects. Antihistamines compete with histamine for cell receptor sites.

INDICATIONS

Benadryl is used for perennial and seasonal allergic rhinitis (hay fever). It is also used for vasomotor rhinitis, allergic conjunctivitis due to inhalant allergens and foods, and mild, uncomplicated allergic skin manifestations. It is also therapeutically useful for anaphylactic reactions

37

adjunctive to epinephrine and other standard measures after the acute manifestations have been controlled. Benadryl is also useful for active and prophylactic treatment of motion sickness. It has been used for parkinsonism in the elderly patient unable to tolerate more potent agents.

PREPARATIONS

Capsules: 25 mg and 50 mg.

DOSAGE

The usual adult dosage is 50 mg three or four times daily. For children (over 20 lb) the dosage is 12.5–25 mg three or four times daily. For motion sickness prophylaxis, the full daily dose, divided as described above, is recommended with the first dose given 30 minutes prior to the journey.

CONTRAINDICATIONS AND PRECAUTIONS

Not for use in newborn or premature infants; not for use in pregnancy or in asthmatics, when hypersensitivity to the drug is known, or concomitantly with MAO inhibitors.

ADVERSE REACTIONS

Among 2102 patients on Benadryl in the Boston Collaborative Drug Surveillance Program, drowsiness, fatigue and vertigo occurred in 36 patients and represented the highest incidence of any adverse effect. The frequencies of other side effects were respiratory depression (3), dry mouth (3), CNS excitation (2), gastric retention (1), coma (1), and "other" (3). Thickening of bronchial secretions has also been reported. Other adverse effects have occurred but are rare. MAO inhibitors prolong the drying effects of antihistamines.

LITERATURE

Carruthers, SG, et al: Clin Pharmacol Ther 23:375, 1978 (sedative and antihistaminic actions); Lilienfield, LS, et al: Clin

Pharmacol Ther 19:421, 1976 (cough);
Schwartz, JC: Annu Rev Pharmacol Toxicol 17:325, 1977 (central actions).

BENADRYL ELIXIR® (Parke-Davis)
Diphenhydramine HCl

1981:104
1980:106
1979:107

Benadryl is an antihistamine. It has anticholinergic or drying actions, a central antitussive effect, an antiemetic effect and sedative side effects. Antihistamines compete with histamine for cell receptor sites.

INDICATIONS	Benadryl is useful for perennial and seasonal allergic rhinitis (hay fever). It is also used for vasomotor rhinitis, allergic conjunctivitis due to inhalant allergens and foods, and mild, uncomplicated allergic skin manifestations. It is also therapeutically useful for anaphylactic reactions adjunctive to epinephrine and other standard measures after the acute manifestations have been controlled. Benadryl is also useful for active and prophylactic treatment of motion sickness. It has been used for parkinsonism in the elderly patient unable to tolerate more potent agents.
PREPARATIONS	Each 5 ml (teaspoon) of elixir contains 12.5 mg diphenhydramine HCl with 14% alcohol.
DOSAGE	Adults: 50 mg (4 teaspoons) three or four times daily. Children over 20 lb: 1 or 2 teaspoons three to four times daily.
CONTRAINDICATIONS AND PRECAUTIONS	Not for use in newborn or premature infants; not for use in pregnancy or in asthmatics, when hypersensitivity to the drug

39

is known, or concomitantly with MAO inhibitors.

ADVERSE REACTIONS

Among 2102 patients on Benadryl in the Boston Collaborative Drug Surveillance Program, drowsiness, fatigue, and vertigo occurred in 36 patients and represented the highest incidence of any adverse effect. The frequencies of other side effects were respiratory depression (3), dry mouth (3), CNS excitation (2), gastric retention (1), coma (1), and "other" (3). Thickening of bronchial secretions has also been reported. Other adverse effects have occurred but are rare. MAO inhibitors prolong the drying effects of antihistamines.

LITERATURE

Carruthers, SG, et al: Clin Pharmacol Ther 23:375, 1978 (sedative and antihistaminic actions); Lilienfield, LS, et al: Clin Pharmacol Ther 19:421, 1976 (cough); Schwartz, JC: Annu Rev Pharmacol Toxicol 17:325, 1977 (central actions).

BENDECTIN® (Merrell-Dow)   1981:154
Doxylamine succinate   1980:115
Pyridoxine HCl   1979: 85

Bendectin provides the action of the antihistamine, doxylamine, which has antinauseant and antiemetic activity, and pyridoxine HCl which provides vitamine B_6 supplementation to help avoid this deficiency during pregnancy. Studies also indicate that B_6 has an antinauseant activity.

INDICATIONS

Nausea and vomiting only associated with pregnancy which are not responsive to conservative (non-drug) measures and are sufficiently distressing to require drug intervention.

PREPARATIONS

Tablets containing doxylamine succinate 10 mg and pyridoxine HCl 10 mg.

DOSAGE

Two tablets at bedtime. In severe cases or when nausea occurs during the day, one additional tablet in the morning and another in midafternoon.

CONTRAINDICATIONS AND PRECAUTIONS

There are no specific contraindications though caution should be used when pregnant women take medication; they should be warned of potential drowsiness.

ADVERSE REACTIONS

Doxylamine succinate may cause drowsiness, vertigo, nervousness, epigastric distress, headache, palpitation, diarrhea, disorientation, or irritability. Pyridoxine has a low incidence of side effects. Only 1.4% of 643 patients receiving this vitamin reported side effects (mainly minor) in the Boston Collaborative Drug Surveillance Program.

LITERATURE

Peterson, F: FDA Talk Paper. Oct 1, 1979; Shapiro, S, et al: Am J Obstet Gynecol 128:480, 1977; Smithells, RW, Sheppard, S: Teratology 17:31, 1978.

BENTYL® (Merrell-National)
Dicyclomine HCl

1981:102
1980:102
1979:122

Bentyl is an antispasmodic and anticholinergic. It relieves smooth muscle spasm of the gastrointestinal tract.

INDICATIONS

Bentyl is used for the treatment of functional bowel/irritable bowel syndrome and acute enterocolitis. In the syrup form, it is used for the treatment of infant colic.

PREPARATIONS

Capsules: 10 mg; Tablets: 20 mg. Syrup: 5 ml (teaspoon) of syrup contains 10 mg dicyclomine hydrochloride. Injection for intramuscular use: 2 ml ampuls in which each ml contains 10 mg, and in 10 ml vials in which each ml contains 10 mg plus a preservative.

DOSAGE

The usual adult dosage is 1 or 2 (10 mg) capsules or teaspoons of syrup three or four times daily. The 20 mg tablets may be used in adults: 1 tablet three or four times daily. The dosage in children is 1 (10 mg) capsule or teaspoon of syrup three or four times daily. The infant dosage is ½ teaspoon of syrup diluted with equal volume of water three or four times daily. The parenteral form for use in adults is 2 ml (20 mg) every 4–6 hours intramuscularly only. *Not for intravenous use.*

CONTRAINDICATIONS AND PRECAUTIONS

Bentyl should not be used in patients with the following conditions: obstructive uropathy, obstructive diseases of the gastrointestinal tract, paralytic ileus, intestinal atony (in the elderly or debilitated), unstable cardiovascular status in acute hemorrhage, severe ulcerative colitis, myasthenia gravis and toxic megacolon complicating ulcerative colitis. Use cautiously in patients with glaucoma, prostatic hypertrophy, hepatic and renal disease, cardiovascular disease, autonomic neuropathy, hyperthyroidism and hiatal hernia. Caution should also be observed in infants because of rare reports of respiratory symptoms in the age group, 6 weeks of age and under.

ADVERSE REACTIONS	Adverse reactions include those physiologic manifestations that accompany blockade of the parasympathetic nervous system such as dry mouth, anhidrosis, mydriasis, cycloplegia, tachycardia, constipation, dysuria, and acute urinary retention. Other reactions that may occur include headache, nervousness, drowsiness, weakness, dizziness, insomnia, impotence, suppression of lactation, and allergic reactions.
LITERATURE	King, JC, Starkman, NM: West Med 5:356, 1964; Martin, DC, et al: J Clin Pharmacol 11:42, 1971; Matts, SGF: Br J Clin Pract 21:549, 1967.

BENYLIN® COUGH SYRUP (Parke-Davis)
Diphenhydramine HCl
Alcohol

1981:163
1980:141
1979:135

Diphenhydramine HCl is a potent antihistaminic agent that also possesses an antitussive action.

INDICATIONS	Benylin Cough Syrup is indicated as an antitussive for the control of coughs due to colds or allergies.
PREPARATIONS	Each 5 ml of the syrup contains diphenhydramine HCl 12.5 mg and alcohol 5% plus inactive ingredients.
DOSAGE	Adults: 2 teaspoons (10 ml) every 4 hours, not to exceed 12 teaspoons in 24 hours. Children, 6–12 years of age: 1 teaspoon (5 ml) every 4 hours, not to exceed 6 teaspoons in 24 hours; 2–6 years of age: ½

teaspoon (2.5 ml) every 4 hours, not to exceed 3 teaspoons in 24 hours.

CONTRAINDICATIONS
AND PRECAUTIONS

Use in children under 6 years of age requires close supervision of a physician. Not for use for persistent cough due to smoking, asthma, emphysema or when cough is accompanied by excessive secretions. This drug should not be used in patients with epilepsy, glaucoma, difficulty in urination due to enlarged prostate gland unless under the advise and supervision of a physician. Avoid drinking alcoholic beverages or engaging in tasks that require complete mental alertness when taking this drug.

ADVERSE REACTIONS

The most frequent are sedation, sleepiness, dizziness, disturbed coordination, epigastric distress, and thickening of bronchial secretions. Less frequently occurring are disturbances of the cardiovascular, hematologic, and genitourinary systems, and various sensitivity reactions. MAO inhibitors prolong the anticholinergic actions of antihistamines.

LITERATURE

AMA Drug Evaluations, 4th ed. New York, AMA and Wiley, 1980, p. 471.

BRETHINE® (Geigy)
Terbutaline sulfate

1981:107
1980:110
1979:132

Brethine, a synthetic sympathomimetic amine, is an antiasthmatic agent; it acts on the beta-adrenergic receptors which cause relaxation of bronchial smooth muscle. Studies have shown that terbutaline relieves the bronchospasm in chronic and acute obstructive pulmonary disease.

INDICATIONS	Brethine is indicated as a bronchodilator for bronchial asthma and for reversible bronchospasms which may occur in association with bronchitis and emphysema.
PREPARATIONS	Tablets: 2.5 and 5.0 mg. Ampuls: 1.0 mg in 1 ml for subcutaneous injection.
DOSAGE	Adults: 5 mg three times a day (not to exceed 15 mg in a 24 hour period). Children, 12–15 years old: use half the adult dose. The usual subcutaneous dose in adults is 0.25 mg into the lateral deltoid area; a second dose may be given in 15–30 minutes if required (not to exceed 0.5 mg in a four hour period). Not recommended for children under the age of 12 years, pending the outcome of studies in this age group.
CONTRAINDICATIONS AND PRECAUTIONS	In cases of known hypersensitivity to sympathomimetic amines. Use with caution in patients with diabetes, hypertension, hyperthyroidism, and with a history of seizures or cardiac problems. As with any medication, caution should be observed in pregnant patients.
ADVERSE REACTIONS	Nervousness and tremor are commonly seen; others reported are headache, increased heart rate, palpitations, drowsiness, sweating, muscle cramps, nausea, and vomiting.
LITERATURE	Miller, WC, and Rice, DL: Ann Allergy 44:15, 1980; Drugs of choice from the Medical Letter. Medical Letter, pp 5–8, 1979; Bone, RC, and Hiller, C: JACEP 7:269, 1978; Manaligoid, LM, et al: Chest 76:532, 1979; Simons, FER, et al: Ann Allergy 43:275, 1979.

BUTAZOLIDIN® ALKA (Geigy)
Phenylbutazone

1981:81
1980:62
1979:52

Butazolidin is an anti-inflammatory, antipyretic, and analgesic agent, with mild uricosuric properties. The drug produces symptomatic relief only and usually does not alter the disease processes for which it is indicated. Butazolidin should not be considered a simple analgesic that can be prescribed for indiscriminate use. This drug is not a salicylate nor a steroid.

INDICATIONS

The most important uses for phenylbutazone are acute gouty arthritis, active rheumatoid arthritis, active ankylosing spondylitis, painful shoulder, and short-term treatment of acute attacks due to degenerative joint disease of the hips and knees that do not respond to other treatments.

PREPARATIONS

Capsules: phenylbutazone 100 mg, dried aluminum hydroxide gel 100 mg, and magnesium trisilicate 150 mg. *Note: The "Alka" preparation was withdrawn by the company in September, 1981. Presently available as Butazolidin in tablets or capsules each containing 100 mg phenylbutzone.*

DOSAGE

For acute gouty arthritis: initially 400 mg followed by 100 mg every four hours. Not for more than one week. For other conditions: the initial adult dose is 300–600 mg daily given as three to four divided doses. After 1 week the dosage should be reduced to a level necessary to maintain relief, not exceeding 400 mg daily. It is recommended that the drug be taken with milk or with meals to minimize gastric upset.

CONTRAINDICATIONS
AND PRECAUTIONS

Butazolidin is contraindicated in children under 14 years of age and in senile patients. Other contraindications are in patients with incipient heart failure, blood disorders, pancreatitis parotitis, stomatitis, polymyalgia rheumatica, temporal arteritis, drug allergy, severe renal, cardiac, and hepatic diseases, and in patients with a history of peptic ulcer or gastrointestinal inflammation. Use with caution in pregnant and nursing women. Butazolidin is contraindicated in patients with known or suspected toxicity, sensitivity, or idiosyncrasy to phenylbutazone or oxyphenbutazone.

ADVERSE REACTIONS

In the Boston Collaborative Drug Surveillance Program 128 patients received phenylbutazone. Among these the following adverse reactions (in number of patients) were noted: gastrointestinal disturbances (5), gastrointestinal bleeding (2), hot flashes (1), ankle edema (1), leukopenia (1), and prolonged prothrombin time (1). Adverse reactions with phenylbutazone affect many systems but most occur with an incidence of less than 1% (see Sperling, 1969, for a discussion of adverse reactions). Phenylbutazone enhances the actions of oral anticoagulants and oral hypoglycemics and increases methotrexate toxicity.

LITERATURE

Sperling, IL: Lancet 2:535, 1969; Strandberg, B: Acta Rheum Scand (Suppl 10), 1965; Symposium (various authors): J Int Med Res 5 (Suppl 2):2, 1977.

BUTISOL® SODIUM (McNeil)
Sodium butabarbital

1981:147
1980:142
1979:131

Butabarbital is a general depressant of the central nervous system. In ordinary doses the drug acts as a sedative and hypnotic. The onset of action is approximately 30 minutes and the duration of action is 5 to 6 hours.

INDICATIONS

Butisol Sodium is used as a sedative or hypnotic.

PREPARATIONS

Tablets: 15, 30, 50, and 100 mg. Capsules: 15 and 30 mg. Elixir: 30 mg in 5 ml with 7% alcohol.

DOSAGE

For adults as a daytime sedative, 15–30 mg three or four times daily. For bedtime hypnosis or preoperative sedation, 50–100 mg. For daytime sedation in children the dosage range is 7.5–30 mg depending on age and weight. When used at bedtime in children the physician should determine the dose based on age and weight.

CONTRAINDICATIONS
AND PRECAUTIONS

This drug is not for use in patients with known sensitivity to barbiturates or in patients with previous addiction to sedatives/hypnotics. It is contraindicated in patients with porphyria or marked impairment of liver function or with respiratory disease where dyspnea or obstruction is present. This drug should not be administered in the presence of acute pain since paradoxical excitement may occur, nor should it be used in patients with borderline hypoadrenal function. Safe use in pregnant women and nursing mothers has not been established.

Residual sedation or "hangover," drowsiness, and lethargy. Respiratory and/or circulatory collapse can occur as can allergic reactions and nausea and vomiting. This drug may be habit forming. Barbiturates interact with the following: alcohol, oral anticoagulants, tricyclic antidepressants, corticosteroids, digitoxin, meperidine, phenothiazines, quinidine, rifampin, and tetracyclines (see Medical Letter reference for updated list).

LITERATURE AMA Drug Evaluations, 4th ed. New York, AMA and Wiley, 1980, p 152; Medical Letter 23(5):17, 1981.

CATAPRES® (Boehringer Ingelheim)
Clonidine HCl

1981:106
1980:132
1979:133

Catapres is an antihypertensive agent whose mechanism of action appears to be central alpha-adrenergic stimulation resulting in the inhibition of sympathetic outflow.

INDICATIONS Catapres is indicated in the treatment of hypertension. It may be employed in a general treatment program with a diuretic and/or other agent, or it may be used alone.

PREPARATIONS Tablets: 0.1, 0.2, and 0.3 mg.

DOSAGE The usual adult *initial* dose is one 0.1 mg tablet twice daily. Further increments of 0.1 or 0.2 mg per day may be made until a satisfactory response is achieved. The usual range is 0.2–0.8 mg per day in divided doses.

| CONTRAINDICATIONS AND PRECAUTIONS | Not recommended for women who are or may become pregnant. No experience is available on the use of clonidine in children. |

CONTRAINDICATIONS AND PRECAUTIONS

Not recommended for women who are or may become pregnant. No experience is available on the use of clonidine in children.

ADVERSE REACTIONS

Most commonly seen are dry mouth (40%), drowsiness (35%), and sedation (8%). Constipation, dizziness, headache, and fatigue have been reported. Although occurring rarely, clonidine has been associated with reactions involving the cardiovascular, central nervous, and genitourinary systems, and with dermatologic and metabolic problems. A rebound phenomenon consisting of a rapid rise in blood pressure, nervousness, agitation, and headache may occur when the drug is withdrawn; thus, when discontinuing therapy the dose should be gradually reduced over a period of 1–2 weeks. Clonidine's antihypertensive effect may be decreased when tricyclic antidepressants or tolazoline are used. Also, clonidine can decrease the signs of hypoglycemia in patients on oral hypoglycemics; however, this finding may not be clinically significant. (See review by Houston, 1981.)

LITERATURE

Geyskes, GG, et al: Br J Clin Pharmacol 7:55, 1979; Houston, MC, Prog Cardiovasc Dis 23:337, 1981. Lowenstein, J: Ann Intern Med 92:74, 1980; Medical Letter 23:45, 1981; Pettinger, WA: N Engl J Med 293:1179, 1975.

CECLOR® (Lilly)
Cefaclor

1981: 80
1980:123
1979: —

Cefaclor is a semisynthetic cephalosporin antibiotic for oral administration. Like other cephalosporins, cefaclor acts by inhibiting cell wall synthesis and is bactericidal.

In vitro testing and clinical use indicate that cefaclor is effective against *Streptococcus pyogenes* (group A beta-hemolytic), *S. pneumoniae*, *E. coli*, *P. mirabilis*, *Klebsiella* species, and *H. influenzae* (including some ampicillin-resistant strains). Although cephalosporins generally have a greater antibacterial spectrum than penicillins, they should not be regarded as first-choice drugs for presumed infections. These drugs are often prescribed for patients allergic to penicillin, but such patients may also be allergic to cephalosporins.

INDICATIONS	This drug is indicated in the following infections when caused by susceptible strains of the invading microorganisms: otitis media, lower respiratory infections, upper respiratory infections (penicillin is the recommended drug for streptococcal infections), urinary tract infections, and skin infections caused by *S. aureus* and *S. pyogenes*.
PREPARATIONS	Capsules: 250 and 500 mg. Powder for suspension: 125 and 250 mg/5 ml.
DOSAGE	Adults: 250 mg every 8 hours (may be increased to 4 g daily in severe cases). Children: 20–40 mg/kg body weight daily in equally divided doses every 8 hours. (The larger child doses are used for otitis media and serious infections; not to exceed 1 g daily.) The dosage in cases of impaired renal function is unchanged, but caution should be exercised in these cases.

Known sensitivity to cephalosporins is a contraindication. Cephalosporins should be used cautiously in penicillin-sensitive patients and during pregnancy. (Not for use in infants under 1 month of age.)

ADVERSE REACTIONS

In clinical studies in 1493 patients adverse reactions were as follows: gastrointestinal disturbances (2.5%), hypersensitivity (1.5%), eosinophilia (2%), genital pruritis, or vaginitis (less than 1%). Other reactions have been noted relating to the hepatic, renal, and hematopoietic systems, but the causal relationship is uncertain.

LITERATURE

McLinn, SE: Curr Chemother 1:123, 1978; Medical Letter, 21:85, 1979; Medical Letter 24:21, 1982 (choice of antimicrobials); Nelson, JD, et al: Am J Dis Child 132:992, 1978.

CENTRAX® (Parke-Davis)
Prazepam

1981:178
1980: —
1979: —

Prazepam is a benzodiazepine derivative with depressant effects on the central nervous system.

INDICATIONS

Centrax is indicated for the management of anxiety disorders or for the short-term relief of the symptoms of anxiety.

PREPARATIONS

Capsules: 5 mg and 10 mg. Tablets: 10 mg.

DOSAGE

The usual daily dose is 30 mg, given in divided doses. The daily dosage should be adjusted within the range 20 mg to

60 mg in accordance with patient response. In elderly or debilitated patients therapy should be initiated with a divided daily dose of 10 to 15 mg. Centrax may also be administered as a single daily dose at bedtime, initially 20 mg (lower in elderly or debilitated patients) with adjustment as needed.

CONTRAINDICATIONS AND PRECAUTIONS

Centrax is contraindicated in patients with known hypersensitivity to this drug, in patients with acute narrow-angle glaucoma, and in psychiatric patients with psychoses or in which anxiety is not a prominent feature. Patients should not use other CNS depressants simultaneously. This drug should not be used by nursing mothers or patients below the age of 18. Usage during pregnancy should almost always be avoided.

ADVERSE REACTIONS

During clinical trials employing a typical 30 mg divided total daily dosage, side effects (and incidence) were as follows: fatigue (11.6%), dizziness (8.7%), weakness (7.7%), drowsiness (6.8%), lightheadedness (6.8%), and ataxia (5.0%). Less frequently reported were headache, confusion, tremor, vivid dreams, slurred speech, palpitation, stimulation, dry mouth, diaphoresis, and various gastrointestinal complaints. Other side effects included pruritis, transient skin rashes, feet swelling, joint pains, various genitourinary complaints, blurred vision and syncope. The actions of benzodiazepines may be potentiated by barbiturates, narcotics, phenothiazines, MAO inhibitors, or other antidepressants.

LITERATURE

Medical Letter 23:41, 1981 (choice of benzodiazepines).

CHLOR-TRIMETON® (Schering)
Chlorpheniramine maleate

1980:175
1979:127

Chlorpheniramine is an antihistamine and hence antagonizes many characteristic effects of histamine. It has anticholinergic (drying) and sedative effects as well.

INDICATIONS	Perennial and seasonal allergic rhinitis; vasomotor rhinitis; allergic conjunctivitis due to foods and inhalant allergens; mild, allergic skin reactions; amelioration of allergic reactions to blood or plasma; as an adjunct to epinephrine in the treatment of anaphylactic reactions.
PREPARATIONS	Tablets: 12 mg. Ampuls: 1 ml ampuls containing 10 mg/ml and 2 ml ampuls containing 100 mg/ml.
DOSAGE	Dosage should be individualized to the patient's needs, but the usual adult dose is one 12 mg tablet at bedtime or every 8–10 hours during the day. The injectable form is used for amelioration of allergic reactions and is given as a single dose of 10–20 mg. The maximum recommended dose for 24 hours is 40 mg. Note: the concentrated injectable form (100 mg/ml) is not to be used by the intravenous route.
CONTRAINDICATIONS AND PRECAUTIONS	This drug should not be used in newborn or premature infants or in nursing mothers. Antihistamines are also contraindicated in asthma, in patients displaying lower respiratory tract symptoms, and in patients with known sensitivity to antihistamines. Use cautiously in patients with elevated ocular pressure, hyperthyroidism, and cardiovascular disease.

54

Drowsiness is the most common, though its incidence is low. Other possible side effects are those characteristic of antihistamines (see Soleymanikashi and Weiss, 1970). In the Boston Collaborative Drug Surveillance Program 237 patients on chlorpheniramine were studied. Among these drowsiness was observed in 4 patients and urinary retention in 1 patient; these were the only side effects among the group. Systems that can be affected by antihistamines include the respiratory, genitourinary, gastrointestinal, cardiovascular, hematologic, and central nervous, but are very rare in ordinary doses. MAO inhibitors prolong the drying action of antihistamines.

LITERATURE

Pearlman, DS: Drugs 12:258, 1976 (review of antihistamines); Soleymanikashi, Y, and Weiss, NS: Ann Allergy 28:486, 1970.

CHOLEDYL® (Parke-Davis)
Oxtriphylline

1981:190
1980:176
1979:176

Choledyl is a xanthine bronchodilator and, compared to aminophylline, is less irritating to the gastric mucosa, more readily absorbed from the gastrointestinal tract, more stable, and more soluble. Like other xanthines, Choledyl is known to increase the vital capacity that is impaired by bronchospasms and air-trapping.

INDICATIONS

Choledyl is indicated for relief of acute bronchial asthma, and for the reversible bronchial spasms associated with chronic bronchitis and emphysema.

55

PREPARATIONS	Tablets: 100 and 200 mg. Sustained action tablets: 400 and 600 mg. Elixir: 100 mg/5 ml plus alcohol 20%. Pediatric syrup: 50 mg/5 ml.
DOSAGE	The usual dosage is 200 or 300 mg, four times a day. The usual dosage in chldren (2–12 years of age) is 100 mg/60 lb body weight, four times a day. When the pediatric syrup is used in children the dose is 6.2 mg/kg body weight administered every 6 hours. Serum theophylline level determination may be a valuable adjunct to dosage adjustment. Optimal therapeutic levels are 10–20 mcg/ml.
CONTRAINDICATIONS AND PRECAUTIONS	Use cautiously in pregnant and lactating women and in the presence of other xanthine preparations (coffee, tea, cola beverages).
ADVERSE REACTIONS	Gastrointestinal disturbances and palpitations may occur. CNS stimulation has been reported. Among 230 patients on oxtriphylline in the Boston Collaborative Drug Surveillance Program the reported side effects (and number of patients) were as follows: gastrointestinal disturbances (10), tachyarrhythmias (3), and "other" (1).
LITERATURE	Hodgkin, JE, et al: JAMA 232:1243, 1976; Medical Letter 20:69, 1978; Thompson, D, et al: Am Rev Resp Dis 117:185, Apr (Suppl) 1978; Thompson, D, Farmer,

CLINORIL® (Merck Sharp & Dohme)
Sulindac

1981:31
1980:27
1979:18

Clinoril is a nonsteroidal anti-inflammatory drug also possessing analgesic and antipyretic activities. Its mode of action, like that of other nonsteroidal anti-inflammatory agents, is not known.

INDICATIONS

Clinoril is indicated for acute or long-term use in the relief of signs and symptoms of the following: osteoarthritis, rheumatoid arthritis, ankylosing spondylitis, acute painful shoulder, and acute gouty arthritis.

PREPARATIONS

Tablets: 150 and 200 mg.

DOSAGE

In osteoarthritis, rheumatoid arthritis, and ankylosing spondylitis, the recommended starting dosage is 150 mg twice a day. In treating acute painful shoulder and acute gouty arthritis the recommended dosage is 200 mg twice a day with a reduction in dosage after a satisfactory response is achieved (approximately 7 days). This drug should be taken with food.

CONTRAINDICATIONS AND PRECAUTIONS

Clinoril is not to be used in patients allergic to aspirin or other nonsteroidal anti-inflammatory drugs, and in patients with demonstrated hypersensitivity to this product. Use with caution in patients with active peptic ulcer or gastrointestinal disturbances and in patients on oral anticoagulants or oral hypoglycemics. Safe use in pregnant women and in nursing mothers has not been established.

ADVERSE REACTIONS

The most common side effects (greater than 1%) are gastrointestinal, dermatologic, and those on the central nervous system such as dizziness and headache. Tinnitus and edema also occur. Reactions with an incidence of less than 1% include gastritis, peptic ulcer, gastrointestinal bleeding, liver abnormalities, dermatologic effects, vertigo, and hypersensitivity reactions.

LITERATURE

Brogden, RN, et al: Drugs 16:97, 1978; Medical Letter 21:1, 1979.

COGENTIN® (Merck Sharp & Dohme)
Benztropine mesylate

1981:160
1980:186
1979:196

Cogentin is an antiparkinsonism drug; it possesses both anticholinergic and antihistaminic effects, although only the former have been established as therapeutically significant in the management of Parkinson's disease. Its anticholinergic activity resembles that of atropine.

INDICATIONS

Cogentin is useful as an adjunct in the therapy of all forms of parkinsonism. It is also used to control extrapyramidal disorders (except tardive dyskinesia) due to neuroleptic drugs such as phenothiazines.

PREPARATIONS

Tablets: 0.5, 1, and 2 mg. The injectable form for intravenous and intramuscular use contains 1 mg/ml in 2 ml ampuls.

DOSAGE

For postencephalitic and idiopathic parkinsonism the usual daily dose is 1 to 2 mg with a range of 0.5–6 mg orally or parenterally, given either as a single dose or divided, depending on patient response. For treating drug-induced extrapyramidal disorders the recommended dose is 1–4 mg once or twice a day orally or parenterally. The oral form is preferred when patients are able to take oral medication.

CONTRAINDICATIONS AND PRECAUTIONS
Not for use in children under 3 years of age or in patients who have demonstrated hypersensitivity to the drug. Use with caution in older children. Safe use in pregnancy has not been established. Use with caution during hot weather to guard against anhidrosis. When used with phenothiazines or other drugs with anticholinergic effects, patient should report g.i. complaints promptly since paralytic ileus may occur.

ADVERSE REACTIONS
Adverse reactions may be anticholinergic or antihistaminic in nature. Dry mouth, blurred vision, nausea, and nervousness may develop. Vomiting occurs but infrequently. Other side effects include constipation, numbness of the fingers, listlessness, and depression. Occasionally allergic reactions develop.

LITERATURE
Medical Letter 21:37, 1979 (drugs for parkinsonism).

COMBID® (Smith Kline & French)
Prochlorperazine maleate
Isopropamide iodide

1981:131
1980:127
1979:114

Combid is broadly classified as a parasympatholytic agent. The prochlorperazine is so prepared that an initial dose is released promptly and the remaining medication is released gradually. The isopropamide iodide component is not in sustained-release form because it can provide 10–12 hours of antisecretory and antispasmodic action. The actions include the reduction of gastric secretion, inhibition of spasm and motility, relief of anxiety and tension, and the control of nausea and vomiting.

INDICATIONS	Possibly effective as adjunctive therapy in peptic ulcer, and in the irritable colon, spastic colon, mucous colitis, functional gastrointestinal disorders, and in functional diarrhea.
PREPARATIONS	Spansule capsules: 10 mg of prochlorperazine, as the maleate, and 5 mg isopropamide iodide equivalent to 5 mg of isopropamide.
DOSAGE	The usual dosage for adults and children over 12 is 1 capsule every 12 hours.
CONTRAINDICATIONS AND PRECAUTIONS	This drug should not be used in children under 12 years of age or in patients with existing drug-induced CNS depression, glaucoma, pyloric obstruction, prostatic hypertrophy, bladder-neck obstruction, obstructive intestinal lesions and/or ileus, bone marrow depression, jaundice, hepatic disease, blood dyscrasias, or in patients with known hypersensitivity.
ADVERSE REACTIONS	The untoward effects are those associated with the components of Combid. Isopropamide may cause dry mouth, urinary hesitancy, tachycardia, palpitations, mydriasis, cycloplegia, blurred vision, constipation, nausea, dysphagia, fever, and nasal congestion. Prochlorperazine may cause drowsiness and confusion, extrapyramidal reactions, CNS excitation, and (rarely) seizures. Respiratory depression and hepatotoxicity may also occur but are very rare.
LITERATURE	AMA Drug Evaluations. New York, AMA and Wiley, 1980, Chapter 61; Ivey, KJ:

Gastroenterology 68:154, 1975 (review of anticholinergics).

COMPAZINE® (Smith Kline & French)
Prochlorperazine

1981:128
1980:107
1979:104

Compazine is one of the class of phenothiazines. These are broadly grouped as antipsychotic and neuroleptics and have effects at all levels of the nervous system. Although the precise mechanisms are unknown, these agents may owe many of their behavioral and neurologic effects to their ability to block dopamine. Phenothiazines have a protective action against nausea and vomiting that is probably related to their dopamine blocking action in the chemoreceptor trigger zone of the medulla.

INDICATIONS

In the management of psychoneurotic patients displaying primarily symptoms of moderate or severe anxiety or tension. It is of questionable value as an antipsychotic agent. An important use is in the control of severe nausea and vomiting. The effectiveness of Compazine in the management of behavioral complications in mentally retarded patients is doubtful.

PREPARATIONS

Tablets: 5, 10, and 25 mg. Capsules: 10, 15, 30, and 75 mg. Ampuls: 2 ml containing 5 mg/ml. Vials: 10 ml containing 5 mg/ml. Disposable syringes: 2 ml containing 5 mg/ml. Suppositories: 2.5, 5, and 25 mg. Syrup: 5 mg/5 ml. Concentrate (for institutional use): 10 mg/ml.

DOSAGE

To treat severe nausea and vomiting or anxiety the usual adult oral dosage is as follows: 5 or 10 mg (tablet form) three or four times daily or by "Spansule" capsule, one 15 mg capsule on arising or one 10 mg capsule every 12 hours. Rectal: 25 mg twice daily in adults. The I.M. dose is 5–10 mg injected deeply into the upper outer quadrant of the buttock. If necessary, repeat in 3–4 hours, not exceeding 40 mg/day. To treat prior to surgery the dosage is 5–10 mg I.M. 1 to 2 hours prior to anesthesia. In adult psychiatry the usual *oral* dosage is 5 to 10 mg three or four times per day. For immediate control in severely disturbed patients an I.M. injection of 10–20 mg into the buttock may be used, repeating if necessary every 2–4 hours. More than 3 or 4 doses are seldom necessary. See package insert for intravenous use. Not for subcutaneous administration.

For use in children (over 20 lb or 2 years of age) the oral and rectal routes are often used, although the intramuscular route is also used. The dosage is based on age, weight, and route. Consult the package insert for details.

CONTRAINDICATIONS AND PRECAUTIONS

Compazine is contraindicated in comatose and greatly depressed states and in the presence of bone marrow depression. Not for use in pediatric surgery, and only with caution during pregnancy. Not for use in children under 2 years of age or under 20 lbs. Use cautiously in children with acute illnesses (e.g., chickenpox, measles, CNS infections, gastroenteritis) or dehydration.

ADVERSE REACTIONS

Drowsiness, dizziness, amenorrhea, blurred vision, skin reactions, and hypotension may occur. Cholestatic jaundice, leukopenia, and agranulocytosis have occurred. In the Boston Collaborative Drug Surveillance Program 1861 patients receiving prochlorperazine were studied.

The side effects (and number of patients experiencing each) were as follows: drowsiness, confusion, or ataxia (13), extrapyramidal reactions (6), CNS excitation (4), seizures (2), repiratory depression (1), and possible hepatotoxicity (1). It is noteworthy that phenothiazines interact with barbiturates, guanethidine, levodopa, lithium, phenytoin, and propranolol.

LITERATURE   Davis, JM, Casper, R: Drugs 14(4):260, 1977; Medical Letter 18(22):89, 1976.

CORGARD® (Squibb)
Nadolol

1981:113
1980: —
1979: —

Nadolol is a synthetic nonselective beta-adrenergic blocking drug. It inhibits both the $beta_1$ receptors located mainly in cardiac muscle and the $beta_2$ receptors located chiefly in the bronchial and vascular musculature. The chronotropic, inotropic and vasodilator responses of beta-adrenergic stimulation are proportionately inhibited. The antihypertensive effects of beta blockers are well known, though the precise mechanism is unknown. (See, for example, INDERAL)

INDICATIONS   Corgard is indicated for the long-term management of patients with angina pectoris. It is also indicated in the management of hypertension, either alone or with other antihypertensives, especially thiazide diuretics.

PREPARATIONS   Tablets: 40, 80, 120, and 160 mg.

DOSAGE   The dosage must be individualized, but the usual ranges are as follows: For angina pectoris—usually 40 mg initially with increments of 40 to 80 mg at 3 to 7 day intervals until optimum clinical response is obtained or there is pronounced slowing of the heart rate. The usual maintenance dose range is 80 to 240 mg administered once daily, with most patients responding to 160 mg per day or less. The safety and usefulness of doses above 240 mg per day for the anginal patient has not been established. For treating hypertension the usual initial adult dose is 40 mg once daily. This dose may be incremented in 40 to 80 mg amounts, gradually until optimal blood pressure reduction is achieved. The maintenance range is usually 80 to 320 mg administered once daily, though in rare cases doses up to 640 daily may be needed. When discontinuing, reduce the daily dosage gradually. Nadolol may be administered without regard to meals.

CONTRAINDICATIONS AND PRECAUTIONS

Nadolol is contraindicated in bronchial asthma, sinus bradycardia and in greater than first degree conduction block, cardiogenic shock, and overt cardiac failure. It is noteworthy that in patients without a history of heart failure, continued use of beta blockers can, in some cases, lead to cardiac failure. Patients with bronchospastic diseases should, in general, not receive beta-blockers. Since withdrawal of beta blockers renders the heart more sensitive to catecholamines, these drugs should be withdrawn *well before surgery* if possible. Beta-adrenergic blockade may prevent the appearance of signs and symptoms of acute hypoglycemia and mask certain signs of hyperthyroidism. Nadolol should be used cautiously in patients with impaired renal or hepatic function and in patients taking catecholamine-depleting drugs such as reserpine. There are no adequate and well-controlled studies on the use of Nadolol in pregnant women; hence, use during pregnancy only if the potential benefit to the mother justifies a potential risk to the fetus. Because it is not known whether this drug is excreted in human milk, it should be used cautiously in nursing women. Safety and effectiveness in children have not been established.

ADVERSE REACTIONS

Bradycardia, with rates below 60 beats per minute is common, and heart rates below 40 beats per minute and/or symptomatic bradycardia were seen in 2 of 100 patients. Symptoms of peripheral vascular insufficiency, usually of the Raynaud type, have occurred in approximately 2 of 100 patients. Cardiac failure, hypotension, and rhythm/conduction disturbances have each occurred in about 1 in 100 patients. Dizziness and fatigue have each been reported in about 2 of 100 patients; paresthesias, sedation, and change in behavior have each been reported in approximately 6 of 1000 patients. Each of the following has been reported in 1 to 5 of 1000 patients: rash, pruritis, headache, dry mouth, eyes or skin, impotence or decreased libido, facial swelling, weight gain, slurred speech, cough, nasal stuffiness, sweating, tinnitus, and blurred vision. Potential adverse effects are those that have been reported with beta blockers (See package insert).

LITERATURE

Medical Letter 22:33, 1980 (review).

CORTISPORIN® OTIC (Burroughs Wellcome)

1981:88
1980:81
1979:89

Polymyxin B
Neomycin
Hydrocortisone

Hydrocortisone, an adrenal corticosteroid, has antiallergic antipruritic and anti-inflammatory activity. Polymyxin B is one of a group of closely related substances produced by various strains of *Bacillus polymyxa*. Its activity is restricted to gram-negative bacteria. Neomycin has antibacterial activity in vitro against the wide range of both gram-negative and gram-positive organisms, with effectiveness against many strains of *Proteus*.

INDICATIONS	For the treatment of superficial infections of the external auditory canal caused by organisms susceptible to the action of the antibiotics. The suspension is used also for treating infections of mastoidectomy caused by organisms susceptible to the antibiotic.
PREPARATIONS	Solution and suspension: each ml of each contains polymyxin B sulfate 10,000 units, neomycin sulfate 5 mg, and hydrocortisone 10 mg.
DOSAGE	For adults 3 or 4 drops of the solution or the suspension should be instilled into the affected ear three or four times daily. For infants and children 3 drops are suggested.
CONTRAINDICATIONS AND PRECAUTIONS	This product is contraindicated in herpes simplex, vaccinia, varicella, and in patients with known sensitivity to any of its components.
ADVERSE REACTIONS	Neomycin may cause cutaneous sensitization. Stinging and burning may occur when the drug reaches the middle ear.

LITERATURE   Glassman, JM, et al: Curr Ther Res
                  23(5):SS29, 1978; Nakamura, T, et al:
                  EENT Monthly 51(4):148, 1972; Ordo-
                  nez, GE: Curr Ther Res 23(5):SS3, 1978.

COUMADIN® (Endo)   **1981:95**
Crystalline warfarin sodium   **1980:92**
                                                  1979:90

Coumadin is an oral anticoagulant that acts by depressing the synthesis in the liver of several clotting factors that are known to be active
in the coagulation mechanism in a variety of diseases characterized
by thromboembolic phenomena. The resulting effect is a sequential
depression of factors II, VII, IX, and X. The degree of depression
is dose related. Oral anticoagulants display different pharmacokinetic
properties and toxicity, and because of these differences, warfarin
sodium is the drug of choice.

INDICATIONS   Coumadin is indicated for prophylaxis
                  and treatment of venous thrombosis and
                  its extension, the treatment of atrial fibril-
                  lation with embolization, the prophylaxis
                  and treatment of pulmonary embolism,
                  and as an adjunct in the treatment of coro-
                  nary occlusion. Coumadin is possibly ef-
                  fective as an adjunct in the treatment of
                  transient cerebral ischemic attacks.

PREPARATIONS   Tablets: 2, 2.5, 5, 7.5, and 10 mg. Vials
                  for injection: 50 mg (I.V. or I.M.)

DOSAGE   Administration and dosage should be
                  gauged according to prothrombin time in
                  the individual patient. Induction may be
                  initiated with 10–15 mg daily and after
                  2 or 3 days adjusted. Most patients are
                  adequately maintained at 2–10 mg daily.
                  The duration of therapy is individualized
                  to the patient's needs.

Anticoagulation is contraindicated in any localized or general physical condition in which there is the possibility of hemorrhage. It is also contraindicated in pregnancy, in conditions in which surgery has been performed or is contemplated, and in cases of active ulceration with bleeding. It should be used cautiously in hypertensive patients, in patients with infectious diseases and in nursing mothers. (See package insert for additional precautions.)

ADVERSE REACTIONS

Hemorrhage is the most common reaction. In the Boston Collaborative Drug Surveillance Program 1029 patients on warfarin sodium were studied. Bleeding reactions occurred in 55 patients (7 serious) and excessive prothrombin time occurred in 28 patients. There was 1 case of rash, 1 case of shock, and 3 reactions listed as "other." Oral anticoagulants interact with a large number of other drugs (see Medical Letter reference).

LITERATURE

Brozovic, M: Semin Hematol 15:27, 1978; Hull, JH, et al: Clin Pharmacol Ther 24(6):644, 1978; Medical Letter 23(5):17, 1981; O'Reilley, RA, Aggeler, PM: Pharmacol Rev 22:35, 1970; Wessler, S: Am J Med Sci 274:106, 1977.

CYCLOSPASMOL® (Ives)
Cyclandelate

1981:188
1980: —
1979: —

Cyclospasmol is an orally acting vasodilator.

INDICATIONS	Adjunctive therapy in intermittent claudication; arteriosclerosis obliterans: thrombophlebitis (to control associated vasospasm and muscular ischemia); nocturnal leg cramps; Raynaud's phenomenon; and for selected cases of ischemic cerebral vascular disease.
PREPARATIONS	Capsules: 200 mg and 400 mg. Tablets: 100 mg.
DOSAGE	Initial therapy is in higher doses, that is, 1200 to 1600 mg daily in divided doses before meals and at bedtime. When a clinical response is noted, the dosage can be decreased in 200 mg decrements until a maintenance dose is reached, usually in the range 400 to 800 mg per day in divided doses. Short-term use is rarely beneficial.
CONTRAINDICATIONS AND PRECAUTIONS	This drug is contraindicated in patients with known hypersensitivity to the drug. Cyclandelate should be used with extreme caution in patients with severe obliterative coronary artery or cerebral-vascular disease. The safety of cyclandelate for use during pregnancy and lactation has not been established. Since this drug is a vasodilator, its use in patients having glaucoma requires extreme caution.
ADVERSE REACTIONS	Gastrointestinal distress, usually mild, may occur with Cyclospasmol. These symptoms can often be relieved by taking the drug with meals or by the concomitant use of antacids. Mild flush, headache, feeling of weakness, or tachycardia may occur, especially during the first weeks of administration.
LITERATURE	Capote, B et al: J Am Geriatr Soc 26:360, 1978; Rao, DB et al: J Am Geriatr Soc

25:548, 1977; Sourander, L et al: Angiology 29:133, 1978.

DALMANE® (Roche)
Flurazepam HCl

1981:12
1980:12
1979:10

Flurazepam is a member of the class of benzodiazepine sedative hypnotics. It is used for the treatment of insomnia.

INDICATIONS	Dalmane is a hypnotic sedative agent used in all types of insomnia characterized by difficulty in falling asleep, frequent nocturnal awakenings, and/or early morning awakenings. Dalmane can be used effectively in patients with recurring insomnia or poor sleeping habits, and in acute or chronic medical situations that require restful sleep.
PREPARATIONS	Capsules: 15 and 30 mg.
DOSAGE	The usual adult dosage is 30 mg before retiring. In some (especially elderly and/or debilitated) patients 15 mg may be sufficient.
CONTRAINDICATIONS AND PRECAUTIONS	Dalmane is contraindicated in patients with known sensitivity to the drug. Alcohol and other CNS depressants must be taken cautiously during use of Dalmane. Usage during pregnancy is not recommended and the drug should not be used for children under 15 years of age.
ADVERSE REACTIONS	Drowsiness and dizziness may occur, and a number of other reactions have been reported. These include, gastrointestinal disturbances, nervousness and weakness,

palpitations, chest pains, body and joint pains, and genitourinary problems. Other reactions have been reported rarely. Among 1966 patients studied in the Boston Collaborative Drug Surveillance Program side effects were as follows: drowsiness (2.3%), confusion (0.7%), ataxia or vertigo (0.2%), nightmares, hallucinations, insomnia, or agitation (0.2%), sensitivity reactions (0.1%), and gastrointestinal disturbances (0.2%).

LITERATURE

Greenblatt, DJ, et al: Clin Pharmacol Ther 17:1, 1975; Kales, A, et al: Clin Pharmacol Ther 18:356, 1975; Kales, A: JAMA 241:1692, 1979; Medical Letter 23:41, 1981 (choice of benzodiazepines).

DARVOCET-N® 100 (Lilly)
Propoxyphene napsylate
Acetaminophen

1981:20
1980:17
1979:13

Propoxyphene is a mild analgesic. Acetaminophen is an analgesic and antipyretic. Its intrinsic activity for mediating these effects is approximately that of aspirin. It is thus an effective alternative to aspirin, but, unlike aspirin, acetaminophen has only weak anti-inflammatory activity.

INDICATIONS

The use of Darvocet-N 100 is for relief of mild to moderate pain either when the pain is present alone or when it is accompanied by fever.

PREPARATIONS

Tablets: 100 mg propoxyphene napsylate and 650 mg acetaminophen.

DOSAGE

The usual adult dosage is 1 tablet every 4 hours as needed for pain. (Not for use in children.)

71

This drug should not be used in patients with known hypersensitivity to propoxyphene, acetaminophen, or aspirin, or in patients who are suicidal or addiction prone. Use cautiously in patients taking antidepressants, tranquilizers, or alcohol. Safe use in pregnancy has not been established.

ADVERSE REACTIONS

The side effects are those associated with the components. The Boston Collaborative Drug Surveillance Program followed 1215 patients on acetaminophen and found adverse reactions in 4. In the same program, 2828 patients on propoxyphene hydrochloride revealed side effects in 19. The most frequently reported side effects are dizziness, sedation, nausea, and vomiting. Others reported are gastrointestinal and CNS disturbances, headache, weakness, visual problems, and liver dysfunctions. The CNS depressant effect of propoxyphene is additive with that of other CNS depressants. It also interacts with carbamazine and curariform drugs (see Medical Letter reference). The preparation may produce dependence in high doses.

LITERATURE

Jaffe, JH, Martin, WR: In Pharmacological Basis of Therapeutics, 6th ed. (Gilman, AG, Goodman, LS, Gilman, A, eds). New York, Macmillan, 1980, pp 520–521; Medical Letter 23:17, 1981.

DARVON COMPOUND-65 (Lilly)

Propoxyphene HCl
Aspirin
Phenacetin
Caffeine

1981:85
1980:68
1979:55

Propoxyphene is a mild analgesic structurally related to the narcotic analgesic methadone. Aspirin (acetylsalicylic acid) is a well-known analgesic-antipyretic and anti-inflammatory agent with less analgesic intrinsic activity than opioids. Caffeine stimulates the central nervous system and is believed to elevate mood. Phenacetin is an analgesic-antipyretic.

INDICATIONS	Relief for mild to moderate pain.
PREPARATIONS	"Pulvules": propoxyphene HCl 65 mg, aspirin 227 mg, phenacetin 162 mg, and caffeine 32.4 mg.
DOSAGE	The usual adult dosage is 1 pulvule every 4 hours as needed for pain. (Not recommended for children.) The dose should not be exceeded.
CONTRAINDICATIONS AND PRECAUTIONS	This drug is contraindicated in patients with known sensitivity to any one of its components. It is also not for patients who are suicidal or addiction-prone. It should be used cautiously in patients taking antidepressants, tranquilizers, or alcohol. Safe use in pregnancy has not been established.
ADVERSE REACTIONS	In the Boston Collaborative Drug Surveillance Program 641 patients on Darvon Compound (propoxyphene 32 or 65 mg) were followed. Of these 11 patients experienced reactions as follows: gastrointestinal disturbances (7), wheezing (1), minor gastrointestinal bleeding (1), headache

(1), and drowsiness (1). Other adverse reactions have been reported including constipation, abdominal pain, skin rashes, CNS disturbances, and weakness. The phenacetin component of Darvon Compound and Darvon Compound-65 has been associated with severe kidney disease and with cancer of the kidney. Drug interactions with propoxyphene can occur (see Medical Letter reference).

LITERATURE

Jaffe, JH, Martin, WR: In Pharmacological Basis of Therapeutics, 6th ed (Gilman, AG, Goodman, LS, Gilman, A, eds). New York, Macmillan, 1980, pp 520–521; Medical Letter 23:17, 1981.

DEMULEN-21® (Searle)
Ethynodiol diacetate
Ethinyl estradiol

1981:129
1980:112
1979:112

Demulen-21 is a combination oral contraceptive preparation. It acts mainly through the mechanism of gonadotropin suppression due to the estrogenic and progestational activity of the constituents. The predominant effect of estrogen is to inhibit secretion of FSH, while continued action of progesterone (related, but not equated to progestins) is to inhibit LH. Alterations in the genital tract, such as changes in the cervical mucus and the endometrium, may also contribute to the contraceptive effectiveness.

INDICATIONS

For the prevention of pregnancy in women who elect to use oral contraceptives as a method of contraception.

PREPARATIONS

Tablets containing ethynodiol diacetate 1 mg and ethinyl estradiol 50 mcg.

DOSAGE

Two schedules may be used. #1 *Sunday Start.* One tablet daily starting on the first Sunday after the onset of menstruation. (If the period begins on Sunday the patient takes her first tablet that same day.) The last (21st) tablet is taken on a Saturday. The next cycle begins on the Sunday, 8 days after the last pill of the previous cycle was taken. All subsequent cycles will also begin on Sunday. #2 *Day 5 Start.* One tablet daily starting on day 5 of her menstrual cycle (the first day of menstruation is counted as day 1) and continues for 21 days. Subsequent cycles begin on the eighth day after taking her last tablet, again starting on the same day of the week on which she began her first course. All subsequent cycles will begin on that same day of the week, that is one tablet each day for 3 weeks followed by a week of no pill taking.

CONTRAINDICATIONS AND PRECAUTIONS

Oral contraceptives should not be used in women with any of the following conditions: (1) Thrombophlebitis or thromboembolic disorders. (2) A past history of deep vein thrombophlebitis or thromboembolic disorders. (3) Cerebral vascular or coronary artery disease. (4) Known or suspected carcinoma of the breast. (5) Known or suspected estrogen-dependent neoplasia. (6) Undiagnosed, abnormal genital bleeding. (7) Known or suspected pregnancy. (8) Benign or malignant liver tumor which developed during the use of oral contraceptives or other estrogen-containing products.

ADVERSE REACTIONS

A variety of major and minor side effects have been attributed to the use of oral contraceptives. Of major concern are cardiovascular side effects and the induction or promotion of tumors. Cigarette smoking increases the risk of serious cardiovascular side effects from oral contraceptives and the risk increases with age and with heavy smoking.

An increased risk of the following serious adverse reactions has been associated with the use of oral contraceptives: thrombophlebitis, pulmonary embolism, coronary thrombosis, cerebral thrombosis, cerebral hemorrhage, hypertension, gallbladder disease, liver tumors, congenital anomalies.

There is evidence of an association between the following conditions and the use of oral contraceptives, although additional confirmatory studies are needed: mesenteric thrombosis, neuro-ocular lesions, e.g., retinal thrombosis and optic neuritis. The following adverse reactions have been reported in patients receiving oral contraceptives and are believed to be drug-related:

Nausea and/or vomiting, usually the most common adverse reactions, occur in approximately 10% or less of patients during the first cycle. Other reactions, as a general rule, are seen much less frequently or only occasionally. Gastrointestinal symptoms (such as abdominal cramps and bloating), breakthrough bleeding, spotting, change in menstrual flow, dysmenorrhea, amenorrhea during and after treatment, temporary infertility after discontinuance of treatment, edema, chloasma or melasma which may persist, breast changes: tenderness, enlargement, and secretion, change in weight (increase or decrease), change in cervical erosion and cervical secretion, possible diminution in lactation when given immediately postpartum, cholestatic jaundice, migraine, increase in size of uterine leiomyomata, rash (allergic), mental depression, reduced tolerance to carbohydrates, vaginal candidiasis, change in corneal curvature (steepening), intolerance to contact lenses.

The following adverse reactions have been reported in users of oral contraceptives, and the association has been neither confirmed nor refuted: Premenstrual-like syndrome, cataracts, changes in libido, chorea, changes in appetite, cystitis-like syndrome, headache, nervousness, dizziness, hirsutism, loss of scalp hair, erythema multiforme, erythema nodosum, hemorrhagic eruption, vaginitis, porphyria, impaired renal function.

The extensive use of oral contraceptives among women throughout the world has prompted many studies aimed at determining toxicity and other effects of these agents. The data have, in some cases, proved to be convincing whereas in others the associations between the drugs and the reactions have been neither confirmed nor refuted. The literature citation below gives a balanced summary and contains further references.

LITERATURE

Murad, F, Haynes, RC, Jr: In The Pharmacological Basis of Therapeutics, 6th ed (Gilman, AG, Goodman, LS, Gilman, A, eds). New York, Macmillan, 1980, Chapter 61.

DIABINESE® (Pfizer)
Chlorpropamide

1981:35
1980:39
1979:46

Chlorpropamide is an oral hypoglycemic agent; it is *not* an oral form of insulin, but is a member of the sulfonylureas. Its mode of action is believed to be that of stimulation and release of endogenous insulin.

INDICATIONS	Chlorpropamide is used in treating uncomplicated diabetes mellitus in the stable, mild, or moderately severe nonketotic maturity-onset type which cannot be completely controlled by diet alone. It may also be of value in controlling patients who do not respond adequately to other sulfonylurea agents.
PREPARATIONS	Tablets: 100 and 250 mg.
DOSAGE	The usual starting dose in moderately severe, middle-aged, stable diabetic patients is 250 mg daily, whereas older patients should start on daily doses in the range 100–125 mg daily. Maintenance therapy is usually 250 mg daily, but 100 mg may be sufficient in some. Severe diabetics who do not respond to 500 mg/day will usually not respond to higher doses. The total daily dose is usually taken at a single time each morning with breakfast.
CONTRAINDICATIONS AND PRECAUTIONS	Diabinese is not indicated in patients with juvenile diabetes mellitus, severe or unstable "brittle" diabetes, diabetes complicated by ketosis and acidosis, diabetic coma, major surgery, severe infection, or severe trauma. This drug is also contraindicated in pregnant women and in patients with seriously impaired renal, hepatic, or thyroid function.

Side effects with chlorpropamide are higher than with tolbutamide. Hypersensitivity reactions and jaundice may occur. Other reactions include diarrhea, blood dyscrasias, phototoxicity, and edema. Hypoglycemia, although really an exaggeration of the drug's action, can occur especially when the dosage exceeds the patient's requirements. When hypoglycemia occurs the patient should be closely supervised for 3–5 days because of the prolonged action of this drug. The Boston Colaborative Drug Surveillance Program followed 367 patients on chlorpropamide. They found 7 patients with adverse effects as follows: hypoglycemia (5), coma (1), and diarrhea (1). Oral hypoglycemics interact with a number of other drugs (see Medical Letter reference).

LITERATURE Ellenberg, M: Medical Challenge 10(5): May, 1978; Medical Letter 23:17, 1981; Shuman, CR: In Diabetes in Theory and in Practice (symposium, AMA meeting, Dec 1977). Drug Therapy, 1978.

DIGOXIN

1981:55
1980:61
1979:57

Digitalis glycosides, such as digoxin, increase the calcium pool needed for contraction, probably by the inhibition of Na-K-ATPase. Both the force and the velocity of myocardial contraction are increased, and the duration of systole is shortened. The refractory period of the A-V junction is increased, thereby slowing the transmission of impulses between atrium and ventricle.

INDICATIONS Digoxin is useful in congestive failure, especially "low output" failure, as it increases force of myocardial contraction and increases cardiac efficiency. It also increases the refractory period of the A-V node and, thus, is useful in atrial flutter and fibrillation since it slows the ventricular rate that would normally accompany these arrhythmias. (Not indicated in sinus tachycardia unless it is due to failure.)

PREPARATIONS

Tablets: 0.125, 0.25, 0.50 mg. Elixir pediatric: 0.05 mg/ml for oral use; for injection: 2 ml ampuls each containing 0.5 mg; pediatric injections, 0.1 mg in 1 ml ampuls; 1 and 2 ml containers as 0.25 mg/ml.

DOSAGE

Initial dose for adults and children (10 years or older) is 0.75–1.5 mg; average oral maintenance dose is 0.125–0.5 mg daily. In the elderly patient, 0.125–0.25 mg is used for daily maintenance. For intravenous use in adults, 0.5–1 mg in two or three divided doses for digitalization; maintenance is 0.125–0.5 mg daily. Patients with renal insufficiency require smaller than usual maintenance doses.

CONTRAINDICATIONS AND PRECAUTIONS

The presence of toxic effects (see below) induced by any digitalis glycoside is a contraindication for digoxin use.

ADVERSE REACTIONS

Arrhythmias or conduction disturbances, especially ventricular premature beats, are common. A-V block has also been seen. Gastrointestinal disturbances, such as anorexia, nausea, vomiting, and diarrhea, are common. Central nervous system disturbances such as blurred vision, yellow vision, headache, and apathy are also seen. Among 3828 patients on digoxin observed in the Boston Collaborative Drug Surveillance Program 476 has adverse reactions as follows: arrhythmias or conduction problems (327), gastrointestinal disturbances (119), CNS toxicity (4), gynecomastia (4), injection site (I.M.) complications (3), electrolyte disturbances (5), and "other" (14). Digitalis effects are enhanced by certain diuretics and antagonized by certain oral antacids and by sulfosalazine and neomycin. In patients with hypokalemia, toxicity may occur even with serum concentrations of digoxin in the "normal range." Quinidine causes a rise in serum digoxin concentrations with the implication that digitalis toxicity might result.

LITERATURE
Aronson, JK: Clin Pharmacokinet 5(2):137, 1980; Drug Therapy 8:1, 1974; Fisch, C, Surawicz, B: Digitalis. New York, Grune and Stratton, 1969; Johnston, GD, et al: Eur J Clin Pharmacol 16:229, 1979; Marcus, FI: Mod Concepts Cardiovasc Dis 45:77, 1976; Smith, TW, Haber, E: Digitalis (4 parts). N Engl J Med 289:945, 1010, 1063, 1125, 1973.

DILANTIN® SODIUM (Parke-Davis)
Phenytoin sodium

1981:34
1980:35
1979:32

Phenytoin, chemically related to the barbiturates, is an anticonvulsant drug. Its site of action is the motor cortex where the spread of seizure activity is inhibited by the drug; this is accomplished possibly by promoting sodium efflux from neurons, hence stabilizing the threshold against hyperexcitability caused by excessive stimulation or environmental changes that are capable of reducing the membrane sodium gradient.

INDICATIONS
The oral form of Dilantin is useful for the control of grand mal and psychomotor

81

seizures. The parenteral form (injectable form) is indicated for the control of status epilepticus of the grand mal type and for the prevention and treatment of seizures occurring during neurosurgery.

PREPARATIONS

Capsules: 30 and 100 mg. Oral suspensions: 125 mg/5 ml and 30 mg/5 ml (pediatric form). Ampuls: 2 ml containing 50 mg/ml, and 5 ml containing 50 mg/ml. Disposable syringe: 2 ml containing 50 mg/ml. Pediatric forms include 50 mg flavored tablets.

DOSAGE

The oral dosage in adults starting on this drug for grand mal and psychomotor seizures is one 100 mg capsule three times daily, with adjustment if necessary up to 6 capsules daily. The initial pediatric oral dosage is 5 mg/kg/day in two or three equally divided doses with adjustment up to a maximum daily dose of 300 mg. The usual maintenance dose in children is 4–8 mg/kg daily. The parenteral form is used for the control of status epilepticus of the grand mal type and for the prevention of seizures during neurosurgery. For status epilepticus the dose is 150–250 mg given *slowly* intravenously, then 100–150 mg 30 minutes later if necessary. Dosage in children is determined according to body weight in proportion to the dosage for a 150 lb adult. The neurosurgical prophylactic dose is 100 to 200 mg (I.M.) at 4 hour intervals during surgery and continued during the postoperative period. (Consult package insert for further details.)

CONTRAINDICATIONS
AND PRECAUTIONS

Phenytoin is contraindicated in patients with known hypersensitivity. The parenteral form is contraindicated in sinus bradycardia, in cases of heart block, and in patients with Adams-Stokes syndrome. Note: withdrawal or dosage reduction should be done gradually.

ADVERSE REACTIONS

The Boston Collaborative Drug Surveillance Program reports on 920 patients receiving Dilantin. Of these 57 patients experienced adverse reactions as follows: CNS symptoms consisting of drowsiness, ataxia, visual problems, and dysarthria (23), sensitivity reactions (14), hematologic reactions (8), gastrointestinal disturbances (5), injection site complications (2), cardiac arrhythmias (2), and "other" (3).

Gingival hyperplasia occurs frequently. There have also been reports of polyarthropathy, hirsutism, hyperglycemia, and serious cases of toxic hepatitis, liver damage, and periarteritis nodosa. Phenytoin interacts with a number of other drugs (see Medical Letter, 1981, reference).

LITERATURE

Ludden, TM, et al: Clin Pharmacol Ther 21:287, 1977; Medical Letter 21:25, 1979; Medical Letter 23:17, 1981; Symposium: Antiepileptic Drugs. (Woodbury, DM, Penry, JK, Schmidt, RP, eds). New York, Raven Press, 1972.

DIMETANE EXPECTORANT® (Robins)

Brompheniramine maleate
Guaifenesin
Phenylephrine HCl
Phenylpropanolamine HCl
Alcohol

1981:174
1980:151
1979:146

Dimetane Expectorant combines widely used ingredients designed for temporary relief of coughing and the complications of allergic states such as seasonal and perennial allergic rhinitis. The combination has the ability to alleviate allergic conditions. The sympathomimetic amines present in Dimetane are indicated for the temporary relief of nasal congestion. Guaifenesin is present as an expectorant.

INDICATIONS	Dimetane is indicated for relief of coughing and the symptomatic relief of many manifestations of allergic states in which expectorant action is desired.
PREPARATIONS	Each 5 ml (1 teaspoon) contains brompheniramine maleate 2 mg, guaifenesin 100 mg, phenylephrine HCl 5 mg, phenylpropanolamine HCl 5 mg, and alcohol 3.5%.
DOSAGE	Adults: 1 to 2 teaspoons four times a day. Children: ½ to 1 teaspoon three to four times a day.
CONTRAINDICATIONS AND PRECAUTIONS	This drug is contraindicated in patients with known sensitivity to any of its ingredients. It should also not be used during pregnancy or lactation, while on MAO inhibitors, and in newborn or premature infants. Use cautiously in patients with narrow angle glaucoma, stenosing peptic ulcer, pyloroduodenal obstruction, prostatic hypertrophy, and bladder-neck obstruction. Not for use in treating lower respiratory tract symptoms including asthma.
ADVERSE REACTIONS	Cardiovascular, hematologic and CNS reactions can occur as well as rashes, anaphylactic shock, photosensitivity, excessive perspiration and dryness. Gastrointestinal, genitourinary and respiratory systems can be affected.
LITERATURE	AMA Drug Evaluations, 4th ed. New York, AMA and Wiley, 1980, pp 470–475; Grater, WC: Arch Otolaryngol 72(1):63,

1960; Irwin, RS: Arch Intern Med 137:1186, 1977; Thomas, JW: Ann Allergy 16:128, 1959.

DIMETAPP® (Robins)
Brompheniramine maleate
Phenylephrine HCl
Phenylpropanolamine HCl

1981:13
1980:10
1979: 9

Dimetapp reduces nasopharyngeal secretions and diminishes inflammatory mucosal edema and congestion in the upper respiratory tract. The antihistamine action of brompheniramine maleate reduces or abolishes the allergic response of nasal tissue. It is complemented by the mild vasoconstrictor action of phenylephrine HCl and phenylpropanolamine HCl which provide a nasal decongestant effect.

INDICATIONS	For the symptomatic treatment of seasonal and perennial allergic rhinitis and vasomotor rhinitis.
PREPARATIONS	Tablets: brompheniramine maleate 12 mg, phenylephrine HCl 15 mg, and phenylpropanolamine 15 mg. Elixir: each 5 ml (1 teaspoon) contains ⅓ the amount in a single tablet plus alcohol 2.3%.
DOSAGE	Adults and children over 12 years of age: 1 tablet morning and evening or 1 to 2 teaspoons three or four times daily. Children, 4 to 12 years of age: 1 teaspoon three or four times daily; 2 to 4 years of age: ¾ teaspoonful three or four times daily; 7 months to 2 years: ½ teaspoonful three or four times daily; 1–6 months; ¼ teaspoonful three or four times daily.
CONTRAINDICATIONS AND PRECAUTIONS	This preparation should not be used during pregnancy and concurrently with

MAO inhibitors. It is also not to be used in treating bronchial asthma. Hypersensitivity to antihistamines of the same chemical class is also a contraindication. The tablets should not be used in children under 12 years of age.

ADVERSE REACTIONS

Hypersensitivity reactions, drowsiness, lassitude, giddiness, dryness of mucous membranes, tightness of chest and thickening of bronchial secretions, urinary frequency and dysuria, cardiovascular symptoms, CNS depression (and occasionally) stimulation, increased irritability, anorexia, nausea, vomiting, and other gastrointestinal disturbances.

LITERATURE

For discussion of the pharmacotherapy of respiratory allergies, see Church, JA, et al: Drug Ther 7:33, 1977; Levine, MI: Compr Ther 4:29, 1978.

DIURIL® (Merck Sharp & Dohme)
Chlorothiazide

1981:94
1980:75
1979:66

Diuril is a diuretic and antihypertensive; it acts by affecting the renal tubular mechanism for electrolyte reabsorption thereby promoting an increase in the excretion of sodium and chloride in approximately equal amounts. Its action is accompanied by a secondary loss of potassium and bicarbonate.

INDICATIONS

Diuril is indicated as adjunctive therapy in edema associated with congestive heart failure, hepatic cirrhosis, and corticosteroid and estrogen therapy. It also has a use in the relief of edema that is associated with various forms of renal dysfunction such as the nephrotic syndrome, acute glomerulonephritis, and chronic renal failure. A very important use of Diuril is in the management of hypertension, either as the sole therapeutic agent, or in combination with other antihypertensive drugs in the more severe cases.

PREPARATIONS

Tablets: 250 mg and 500 mg. Suspension: each 5 ml (1 teaspoon) contains 250 mg chlorothiazide. The intravenous form is a dry white powder in vials containing the salt form equivalent to 0.5 g chlorothiazide.

DOSAGE

For adults the dosage for diuresis is 0.5–1.0 g once or twice a day. For hypertension the (adult) starting dose is 0.5–1.0 g a day either as a single dose or divided. The dosage is then adjusted according to patient response. For infants and children the dosage is based on body weight: 10 mg/lb body weight daily given in two divided doses. The intravenous route is used in emergencies or when the patient cannot take the oral form. The adult dosage is 0.5–1.0 g once or twice a day. (Not for I.M. or S.C. use.)

CONTRAINDICATIONS
AND PRECAUTIONS

Anuria and hypersensitivity to this or other sulfonamide-derived drugs.

ADVERSE REACTIONS

The reported side effects are gastrointestinal, hematologic, cardiovascular, and CNS-related, as well as hypersensitivity reactions and other effects such as hyperglycemia, hypokalemia, hyperuricemia, hyponatremia, and sensitivity reactions. Among 688 patients on chlorothiazide studied in the Boston Collaborative Drug Surveillance Program adverse reactions were experienced by 73 patients as follows: dehydration (42), hypokalemia (11), hyperuricemia (6), sensitivity reactions

(6), hyponatremia (2), hyperglycemia (2), gastrointestinal disturbances (2), and "other" (2).

LITERATURE Kuchel, OG, et al: Can Med Assoc J 120(5):565, 1979 (hypertension); Lief, PD: Am Heart J 96(6):824, 1978 (cardiac therapy); McMahon, FG: *Management of Essential Hypertension.* Mount Kisco, New York, Futura Publishing, 1978, Chapter 2; Medical Letter 23:45, 1981; Morgan, T, et al: Clin Sci Mol Med 55(Suppl 4): 305S, 1978 (hypertension).

DONNATAL® (Robins)   1981:32
Phenobarbital   1980:28
Hyoscyamine sulfate   1979:24
Atropine sulfate
Hyoscine hydrobromide

Donnatal combines several natural belladonna alkaloids with phenobarbital to provide peripheral anticholinergic and antispasmodic action with mild sedation.

INDICATIONS Possibly effective as adjunctive therapy in the treatment of peptic ulcer, in irritable bowel syndrome, and acute enterocolitis.

PREPARATIONS Tablets (regular), No. 2 Tablets, capsules, elixir, and Extentabs. Each (regular) tablet, capsule or 5 ml (1 teaspoon) of elixir (23% alcohol) contains phenobarbital 16.2 mg, hyoscyamine sulfate 0.1037 mg, atropine sulfate 0.0194 mg, and hyoscine hydrobromide 0.0064. Each No. 2 tablet contains 32.4 mg phenobarbital and the same amounts of the other components as above. The Extentab contains the equivalent of three regular tablets and releases the ingredients gradually.

<table>
<tr><td>DOSAGE</td><td>The recommended adult dose is 1 or 2 tablets or capsules three or four times a day, or 1 or 2 teaspoonfuls of elixir three or four times a day depending on the severity of symptoms. The adult dose when No. 2 tablets are used is 1 or 2 No. 2 tablets three times a day. The usual dose for Extentabs is 1 every twelve hours. The elixir is used in children in quantities based on body weight: 10 lb, 0.5 ml; 20 lb, ¼ tsp; 30 lb, ½ tsp; 50 lb, ¾ tsp; 75–80 lb, 1 tsp. These doses may be repeated every 4–6 hours.</td></tr>
<tr><td>CONTRAINDICATIONS AND PRECAUTIONS</td><td>Donnatal is contraindicated in patients with glaucoma, renal, or hepatic disease, obstructive uropathy, or hypersensitivity to any of the ingredients. (Phenobarbital may be habit forming.)</td></tr>
<tr><td>ADVERSE REACTIONS</td><td>Blurred vision, dry mouth, difficult urination, and flushing or dryness of the skin.</td></tr>
<tr><td>LITERATURE</td><td>Ivey, KJ: Gastroenterology 68:154, 1975 (anticholinergics and peptic ulcer); Sleisenger, M, Fordtran, J: Gastrointestinal Disease. Philadelphia, Saunders, 1973. (See also TAGAMET for literature pertinent to this area)</td></tr>
</table>

DRIXORAL® (Schering)
Dexbrompheniramine maleate
Pseudoephedrine sulfate

1981:45
1980:45
1979:56

Drixoral combines the antihistaminic actions of dexbrompheniramine with the vasoconstrictive actions of pseudoephedrine.

89

INDICATIONS	Drixoral is indicated for the relief of symptoms of upper respiratory mucosal congestion in seasonal and perennial allergies, acute rhinitis, acute rhinosinusitis, and eustachian tube blockage.
PREPARATIONS	Tablets (sustained release); dexbrompheniramine maleate 6 mg and pseudoephedrine sulfate 120 mg.
DOSAGE	For adults and children over 12 years: 1 tablet in the morning and 1 at bedtime.
CONTRAINDICATIONS AND PRECAUTIONS	Drixoral is contraindicated in patients with severe hypertension and coronary artery disease. This preparation is not for children under 12 years of age or for pregnant women and nursing mothers.
ADVERSE REACTIONS	The side effects are those associated with sympathomimetic and antihistaminic drugs. These include drowsiness, confusion, restlessness, nausea, vomiting, gastrointestinal symptoms, drug rash, vertigo, anorexia, dizziness, dysuria, headache, insomnia, anxiety, tension, weakness, tachycardia, and other cardiovascular effects.
LITERATURE	Fierberg, AA: Ann Allergy 22:324, 1964; Pearlman, DS: Drugs 12:258, 1976 (review of antihistamines).

DYAZIDE® (Smith Kline & French)
Triamterene
Hydrochlorothiazide

1981:3
1980:4
1979:6

Dyazide is a diuretic/antihypertensive. It combines the diuretic action of triamterene with the diuretic and antihypertensive action of hydrochlorothiazide. Triamterene acts on the distal renal tubule to inhibit the reabsorption of sodium in exchange for potassium and hydrogen ions. Hydrochlorothiazide blocks reabsorption of sodium and chloride ions, thus increasing the quantity of sodium traversing the distal tubule and the volume of water excreted. The continued use of hydrochlorothiazide may lead to excessive loss of potassium, hydrogen, and chloride ions as a compensatory phenomenon. The triamterene component, because of its potassium sparing actions, is useful in combination with the thiazide when treating hypertension.

INDICATIONS	Dyazide is mainly used in the treatment of edema; it is also used to treat hypertension.
PREPARATIONS	Capsules: triamterene 50 mg and hydrochlorothiazide 25 mg.
DOSAGE	The usual adult daily dosage is 1 or 2 capsules twice a day after meals (not to exceed 4 capsules a day). Information on the use of Dyazide in children is inadequate.
CONTRAINDICATIONS AND PRECAUTIONS	Dyazide is contraindicated in cases of anuria or progressive renal dysfunction and in patients who develop hyperkalemia. It is not for use in patients with preexisting elevated serum potassium or hepatic dysfunction. Hypersensitivity to either component of Dyazide or to other sulfonamide-derived drugs is a contraindication. Thiazides cross the placental barrier, hence their use in pregnancy requires that the anticipated benefit be weighed against possible hazards to the fetus. Mothers should not nurse if the use of this drug is deemed essential.
ADVERSE REACTIONS	Muscle cramps, weakness, dizziness, headache, dry mouth, gastrointestinal disturbances, and sensitivity reactions. (See HYDROCHLOROTHIAZIDE.)

LITERATURE   Council on Drugs. JAMA 192(10):853, 1965; Holland, OB, et al: Curr Ther Res 22(4):479, 1977; Medical Letter 7(5):17, 1965; Medical Letter 23:45, 1981; Page, LB, et al: Am Heart J 91(6):810, 1976.

E.E.S.® (Abbott)

Erythromycin ethylsuccinate

1981:19
1980:22
1979:26

Erythromycin, from the macrolide group of antibiotics, inhibits bacterial protein synthesis. It is widely used as an alternate to penicillin and is one of the safest antibiotics currently in use. Besides its use as an alternate to penicillin, erythromycin is the recommended drug in many disease states. It diffuses readily into most body fluids, but only low concentrations are achieved in the spinal fluid. The oral forms are preferred though these are inactivated to varying degrees by gastric juice.

INDICATIONS   Erythromycin is effective in the treatment of infections caused by *S. pyogenes, S. aureus, S. pneumoniae, M. pneumoniae, H. influenza* (concomitant with a sulfonamide), *Treponema pallidum* and *L. monocytogenes.* Erythromycin is used in Legionnaires Disease, chlamydial infections, intestinal amebiases, erythrasma, and as an adjunct to antitoxin in the treatment of diphtheria. Erythromycin is also effective in *Bordetella pertussis* (whooping cough) in eliminating the organism from the nasopharynx of infected individuals and may be used with injectable (lactobionate) forms as an alternate treatment of acute pelvic inflammation caused by *N. gonorrhoeae* in female patients sensitive to penicillin. Injectable penicillin G benzathine is recommended by the American Heart Association in the treatment and prevention of streptococcal pharyngitis and long-term prophylaxis of rheumatic fever. Oral penicillin G or V or erythromycin are alternates in the above conditions. Erythromycin is used by patients with a history of heart disease and who are sensitive to penicillin for short-term prophylaxis prior to dental procedures.

PREPARATIONS

Oral suspension: 200 and 400 mg/5 ml. Granules for oral suspension: 200 mg/5 ml after reconstitution. Drops: 100 mg/2.5 ml (½ teaspoon) after reconstitution. Chewable tablets: 200 mg. Film tab tablets: 400 mg.

DOSAGE

Adults: 400 mg four times daily is the usual dosage. For severe infections in adults 4 g daily in divided doses may be given. Children: 30–50 mg/kg/day in equally divided doses.

CONTRAINDICATIONS AND PRECAUTIONS

Erythromycin should not be used in patients with known hypersensitivity to the drug. Caution should be exercised in patients with impaired hepatic function and those on theophylline therapy. The safety of erythromycin during pregnancy has not been established.

ADVERSE REACTIONS

Erythromycins may cause reversible cholestatic jaundice, but other serious side effects are seldom seen. The main side effects associated with oral erythromycin are mild gastrointestinal disturbances (nausea, vomiting, pyrosis, diarrhea), but these occur infrequently. Sensitivity reactions occur infrequently and sensorineural hearing loss (reversible) has been associated with the use of large doses of erythromycin, but is very rare. Among 375 patients on various forms of erythromycin in the Boston Collaborative Drug Surveillance Program 40 patients had side effects as follows: gastrointestinal disturbances (mainly minor, 24), sensitivity reactions (8), injection site complications (4), super-infection (3), and "other" (1).

Erythromycin can increase the effects of theophylline; the parenteral forms may be incompatible with solutions of vitamin B complex, ascorbic acid, cephalothin, tetracycline, colistin, chloramphenicol, heparin, metaraminol, and phenytoin.

LITERATURE

Lacey, RW: Postgrad Med J 53:195, 1977 (new look at erythromycin); Medical Letter 24:21, 1982 (choice of antimicrobials); Nicholas, P: NY State J Med 77:2088 and 2243, 1977 (clinical pharmacology and therapeutic uses); Olmstead, CB: Cutis 24:414 and 422, 1979 (dermatologic use); Sanford, JP: N Engl J Med 300:654, 1979 (Legionnaire's disease); Symposium (on erythromycin) Scott Med J 22(Suppl. 1): 349, 1977.

ELAVIL® (Merck Sharp & Dohme)
Amitriptyline HCl

1981:42
1980:37
1979:34

Amitriptyline is an antidepressant with antianxiety action and a sedative component. Its precise mechanism is not known; it is not a monoamine oxidase inhibitor and it does not act primarily by stimulating the central nervous system. Amitriptyline is known to inhibit the membrane mechanism responsible for reuptake of norepinephrine into adrenergic neurons.

INDICATIONS

Elavil is used for the relief of symptoms of depression. Endogenous depression is

94

more likely to be alleviated than are other depressive states.

PREPARATIONS

Tablets 10, 25, 50, 75, 100, and 150 mg. Sterile solution for intramuscular injection. Each ml of the solution contains amitriptyline HCl 10 mg, dextrose 44 mg, water for injection, and preservatives.

DOSAGE

The initial daily dosage for adults is 75 mg in divided doses and may be increased to 150 mg if necessary. Alternatively therapy may be initiated with 50–100 mg at bedtime. Lower doses are recommended for adolescent and elderly patients (eg, 10 mg, three times a day, with 20 mg at bedtime). Adequate response may take 30 days to develop. Maintenance dosage is 50–100 mg daily. When therapy is initiated with the parenteral route (I.M.) 20 or 30 mg daily (2–3 ml) four times a day may be used. Elavil is not for patients under 12 years of age.

CONTRAINDICATIONS AND PRECAUTIONS

This drug is contraindicated in patients with known hypersensitivity. Also, it should not be used concomitantly with MAO inhibitors. (Wait 14 days between the last dose of an MAO inhibitor if Elavil is being started.) Elavil is contraindicated during the acute recovery phase following myocardial infarction.

ADVERSE REACTIONS

Adverse reactions include effects on the CNS (drowsiness and confusion), the cardiovascular system, the gastrointestinal system and the hematologic system as well as anticholinergic effects and allergic reactions. Among 309 patients receiving Elavil and followed in the Boston Collaborative Drug Surveillance Program, 40 patients experienced side effects as follows: drowsiness (20), CNS excitation (11), anticholinergic reactions (5), headache or

95

tinnitus (2), and cardiovascular effects consisting of arrhythmias and hypotension (2).

Elavil may block the antihypertensive action of guanethidine and similarly acting drugs, and may enhance the response to alcohol and the effects of barbiturates and other CNS depressants.

LITERATURE

Cecchini, S, et al. J Int Med Res 6:388, 1978; Cutler, NR, Heiser, JF: JAMA 240:2264, 1978; Kampman, R, et al: Acta Psychiatr Scand 58:142, 1978; Klerman, GL, Hirschfeld, RMA: JAMA 240:1403, 1978.

EMPIRIN/CODEINE (Burroughs Wellcome)
Aspirin
Codeine phosphate

1981: 29
1980: 21
1979:109

Aspirin is a non-narcotic analgesic with antipyretic and anti-inflammatory actions. Codeine is a narcotic analgesic with antitussive properties.

INDICATIONS

For the relief of mild to moderately severe pain.

PREPARATIONS

Tablets: Aspirin 325 mg plus codeine phosphate in several different strengths: No. 2—15 mg; No. 3—30 mg; No. 4—60 mg.

DOSAGE

The usual adult dose for No. 2 and No. 3 is one or two tablets every 4 hours as required. The No. 4 tablet is given as one tablet every 4 hours as required.

CONTRAINDICATIONS
AND PRECAUTIONS

Hypersensitivity to aspirin or codeine is a contraindication. This drug should not be used during pregnancy, in the presence of increased intracranial pressure, or in acute abdominal conditions. Use cautiously in elderly and debilitated patients and in patients with impaired renal or hepatic function, hypothyroidism, Addison's disease, prostatic hypertrophy or urethral stricture, peptic ulcer, or coagulation disorders.

ADVERSE REACTIONS

The reactions to codeine affect the gastrointestinal and central nervous systems. In the Boston Collaborative Drug Surveillance Program 817 patients on oral codeine were studied and 29 experienced adverse effects as follows: constipation (14), nausea or vomiting (7), sensitivity reactions (3), vertigo (2), drowsiness (1), hallucinations (1), and coma (1).

The most common side effects of aspirin are headache, vertigo, ringing in the ears, mental confusion, drowsiness, sweating, thirst, and gastrointestinal disturbances that can include gastric bleeding. The CNS depression of codeine can enhance the action of other CNS depressants.

LITERATURE

Cooper, SA, Beaver, WI: Clin Pharmacol Ther 20(2):241, 1976.

E-MYCIN® (Upjohn)
Erythromycin

1981:57
1980:50
1979:63

Erythromycin, from the macrolide group of antibiotics, inhibits bacterial protein synthesis. It is widely used as an alternate to penicillin and is one of the safest antibiotics currently in use. Besides its use as an alternate to penicillin, erythromycin is the recommended drug in many disease states. It diffuses readily into most body fluids, but only low concentrations are achieved in the spinal fluid. The oral forms are preferred though these are inactivated to varying degrees by gastric juice; however, E-Mycin tablets are enteric coated and are not inactivated by the acid milieu of the stomach.

INDICATIONS

Erythromycin is effective in the treatment of infections caused by *S. pyogenes, S. aureus, S. pneumoniae, M. pneumoniae, H. influenza* (concomitant with a sulfonamide), *Treponema pallidum* and *L. monocytogenes*. Erythromycin is used in Legionnaires Disease, chlamydial infections, intestinal amebiases, erythrasma, and as an adjunct to antitoxin in the treatment of diphtheria. Erythromycin is also effective in *Bordetella pertussis* (whooping cough) in eliminating the organism from the nasopharynx of infected individuals and may be used with injectable (lactobionate) forms as an alternate treatment of acute pelvic inflammation caused by *N. gonorrhoeae* in female patients sensitive to penicillin. Injectable penicillin G benzathine is recommended by the American Heart Association in the treatment and prevention of streptococcal pharyngitis and long-term prophylaxis of rheumatic fever. Oral penicillin G or V or erythromycin are alternates in the above conditions. Erythromycin is used by patients with a history of heart disease and who are sensitive to penicillin for short-term prophylaxis prior to dental procedures.

PREPARATIONS

Tablets (enteric coated): 250 mg and 333 mg.

DOSAGE

Adults: 1 g daily in three or four divided doses. Children: 30 to 50 mg/kg body weight daily in three or four divided doses

98

(twice this dose may be used in severe infections). For severe infections in adults 4 g daily in divided doses may be given.

CONTRAINDICATIONS AND PRECAUTIONS

Erythromycin should not be used in patients with known hypersensitivity to the drug. Caution should be exercised in patients with impaired hepatic function and those on theophylline therapy. The safety of erythromycin during pregnancy has not been established.

ADVERSE REACTIONS

Erythromycins seldom cause serious side effects, though the estolate has been reported to cause cholestatic jaundice (more so than other forms). The main side effects associated with oral erythromycin are mild gastrointestinal disturbances (nausea, vomiting, pyrosis, diarrhea), but these occur infrequently. Sensitivity reactions occur infrequently and sensorineural hearing loss (reversible) has been associated with the use of large doses of erythromycin, but is very rare. Among 375 patients on various forms of erythromycin in the Boston Collaborative Drug Surveillance Program 40 patients had side effects as follows: gastrointestinal disturbances (mainly minor, 24), sensitivity reactions (8), injection site complications (4), superinfection (3), and "other" (1).

Erythromycin can increase the serum levels of theophylline.

LITERATURE

Hansten, PD: Drug Interactions Newsletter: 1(2):5, 1981 (theophylline interaction); Lacey, RW: Postgrad Med J 53:195, 1977 (new look at erythromycin); Medical Letter 24:21 (1982) (choice of antimicrobials); Nicholas, P: NY State J Med 77:2088 and 2243, 1977 (clinical pharmacology and therapeutic uses); Olmstead, CB: Cutis 24:414 and 422, 1979 (dermatologic use); Sanford, JP: N Engl J Med 300:654, 1979 (Legionnaire's disease); Symposium (on erythromycin): Scott Med J 22(Suppl 1):349, 1977.

ENDURON® (Abbott) 1981:101
Methyclothiazide 1980:109
 1979:119

Enduron is a diuretic and antihypertensive. Its diuretic and saluretic effects result from drug-induced inhibition of the renal tubular reabsorption of electrolytes. Enduron is structurally related to hydrochlorothiazide.

INDICATIONS Enduron is indicated in the management of hypertension either as the sole therapeutic agent or in combination with other agents to enhance the antihypertensive action of the other agents. Enduron is also indicated as adjunctive therapy in the treatment of various edemas such as those associated with congestive heart failure, hepatic cirrhosis, and corticosteroid and estrogen therapy.

PREPARATIONS Tablets: 2.5 and 5 mg.

DOSAGE The usual adult dosage for edematous conditions ranges from 2.5 to 10 mg once daily. Therapy should be individualized according to patient response. For hypertension the adult dosage range is 2.5–5 mg once daily.

CONTRAINDICATIONS Renal decompensation is a contraindication. Known hypersensitivy to this or other sulfonamide-derived drugs is also a contraindication. Use in pregnant or lactating women is generally not recommended.
AND PRECAUTIONS

ADVERSE REACTIONS	The adverse reactions affect the gastrointestinal system, the central nervous system (dizziness, vertigo, paresthesias, and headache), and the hematologic system. Hypersensitivity reactions also occur. Hypokalemia is a known side effect of thiazide drugs (see Soghikian and Bartenbach, 1977.) Thiazide drugs may increase the responsiveness to tubocurarine and may affect the insulin requirements of diabetic patients. Thiazides also interact with corticosteroids, digitalis drugs, indomethacin, lithium, and salicylates.
LITERATURE	Medical Letter 23:45, 1981; Report of the Joint Medical Committee on High Blood Pressure; JAMA 237(3):255, 1977; Soghikian, K, Bartenbach, DE: South Med J 70:1397, 1977.

EQUAGESIC® (Wyeth)

Meprobamate
Ethoheptazine citrate
Aspirin

1981:142
1980:130
1979:106

Meprobamate has analgesic (and possibly muscle relaxing) actions. When there is musculoskeletal pain it enhances the analgesic effects of other drugs. Ethoheptazine is structurally related to meperidine, but has only mild analgesic activity and extremely low abuse potential. The analgesic, antipyretic, and anti-inflammatory actions of aspirin are well known.

INDICATIONS	Equagesic is possibly effective in the treatment of pain accompanied by tension and anxiety in patients with musculoskeletal disease or tension headache.
PREPARATIONS	Tablets: ethoheptazine citrate 75 mg, aspirin 250 mg, and meprobamate 150 mg.

101

DOSAGE	For adults and children over 12 years of age the usual dosage is 1 or 2 tablets three or four times daily as needed.
CONTRAINDICATIONS AND PRECAUTIONS	Not generally recommended during pregnancy and lactation. Addiction-prone individuals must be carefully supervised.
ADVERSE REACTIONS	Nausea, vomiting, and epigastric distress occur in a small percentage of patients. The meprobamate component may cause drowsiness. Dizziness occurs rarely as do certain allergic reactions and fever. Other allergic reactions have occurred, but are very rare. (See also MEPROBAMATE)
LITERATURE	Scheiner, JJ, Richards, DJ: Curr Ther Res 16(9):928, 1974; Winkelman, NW, Richards, DJ: Curr Ther Res 17(4):352, 1975.

ERYTHROCIN® (Abbott)
Erythromycin stearate and lactobionate

1981:168
1980:147
1979: 96

Erythromycin, from the macrolide group of antibiotics, inhibits bacterial protein synthesis. It is widely used as an alternate to penicillin and is one of the safest antibiotics currently in use. Besides its use as an alternate to penicillin, erythromycin is the recommended drug in many disease states. It diffuses readily into most body fluids, but only low concentrations are achieved in the spinal fluid. The oral forms are preferred though these are inactivated to varying degrees by gastric juice.

INDICATIONS	Erythromycin is effective in the treatment of infections caused by *S. pyogenes, S. aureus, S. pneumoniae, M. pneumoniae, H. influenza* (concomitant with a sulfonamide), *Treponema pallidum* and *L. monocytogenes.* Erythromycin is used in Legionnaires dis-

ease, chlamydial infections, intestinal amebiases, erythrasma, and as an adjunct to antitoxin in the treatment of diphtheria. Erythromycin is also effective in *Bordetella pertussis* (whooping cough) in eliminating the organism from the nasopharynx of infected individuals and may be used with injectable (lactobionate) forms as an alternate treatment of acute pelvic inflammation caused by *N. gonorrhoeae* in female patients sensitive to penicillin. Injectable penicillin G benzathine is recommended by the American Heart Association in the treatment and prevention of streptococcal pharyngitis and long-term prophylaxis of rheumatic fever. Oral penicillin G or V or erythromycin are alternates in the above conditions. Erythromycin is used by patients with a history of heart disease and who are sensitive to penicillin for short-term prophylaxis prior to dental procedures.

PREPARATIONS

Tablets: 125, 250, and 500 mg (as the stearate). Powder (lyophilized): 500 mg and 1 g (as the lactobionate for I.V. use).

DOSAGE

Adults: 250 mg orally every 6 hours or 500 mg every 12 hours given on an empty stomach or immediately before meals. For severe infections in adults 4 g may be given in divided doses. In children, 30–50 mg/kg body weight daily in four divided doses. (For severe infections the dose may be doubled.) When the intravenous route must be used for severe infections in adults and children, 15–20 mg/kg body weight daily. (The maximum dose daily of the lactobionate is 4 g.) Continuous infusion is preferable but administration every 6 hours is also effective.

103

Erythromycin should not be used in patients with known hypersensitivity to the drug. Caution should be exercised in patients with impaired hepatic function and those on theophylline therapy. The safety of erythromycin during pregnancy has not been established.

ADVERSE REACTIONS

Erythromycin may cause reversible cholestatic jaundice but other serious side effects are seldom seen. The main side effects associated with oral erythromycin are mild gastrointestinal disturbances (nausea, vomiting, pyrosis, diarrhea), but these occur infrequently. Sensitivity reactions occur infrequently and reversible hearing loss with doses of 4 g or more per day have been rarely reported. Occasional venous irritation has occurred. Among 375 patients on various forms of erythromycin in the Boston Collaborative Drug Surveillance Program 40 patients had side effects as follows: gastrointestinal disturbances (mainly minor, 24), sensitivity reactions (8), injection site complications (4), superinfection (3), and "other" (1).

Erythromycin can increase the effects of theophylline; the parenteral forms may be incompatible with solutions of vitamin B complex, ascorbic acid, cephalothin, tetracycline, colistin, chloramphenicol, heparin, metaraminol, and phenytoin. No drug or chemical agent should be added to the erythromycin lactobionate IV fluid admixture unless its effect on the chemical and physical stability of the solution has been determined.

LITERATURE

Lacey, RW: Postgrad Med J 53:195, 1977 (new look at erythromycin); Medical Letter 24:21, 1982 (choice of antimicrobials); Nicholas, P: NY State J Med 77:2088 and

2243, 1977 (clinical pharmacology and therapeutic uses); Olmstead, CB: Cutis 24:414 and 422, 1979 (dermatologic use); Sanford, JP: N Engl J Med 300:654, 1979 (Legionnaire's disease); Symposium (on erythromycin): Scott Med J 22(Suppl 1):349, 1977.

ERTHROMYCIN Systemic

1981:21
1980:18
1979:17

Erythromycin, from the macrolide group of antibiotics, inhibits bacterial protein synthesis. It is widely used as an alternate to penicillin and is one of the safest antibiotics currently in use. Besides its use as an alternate to penicillin, erythromycin is the recommended drug in many disease states. It diffuses readily into most body fluids, but only low concentrations are achieved in the spinal fluid. The oral forms are preferred though these are inactivated to varying degrees by gastric juice.

INDICATIONS

Erythromycin is effective in the treatment of infections caused by S. pyogenes, S. aureus, S. pneumoniae, M. pneumoniae, H. influenza (concomitant with a sulfonamide), Treponema pallidum and L. monocytogenes. Erythromycin is used in Legionnaire's disease, chlamydial infections, intestinal amebiases, erythrasma, and as an adjunct to antitoxin in the treatment of diphtheria. Erythromycin is also effective in Bordetella pertussis (whooping cough) in eliminating the organism from the nasopharynx of infected individuals and may be used with injectable (lactobionate) forms as an alternate treatment of acute pelvic inflammation caused by N. gonor-

rhoeae in female patients sensitive to penicillin. Injectable penicillin G benzathine is recommended by the American Heart Association in the treatment and prevention of streptococcal pharyngitis and long-term prophylaxis of rheumatic fever. Oral penicillin G or V or erythromycin are alternates in the above conditions. Erythromycin is used by patients with a history of heart disease and who are sensitve to penicillin for short-term prophylaxis prior to dental procedures.

PREPARATIONS

Tablets: 250 and 500 mg. Enteric coated tablets: 250 mg. (See also E.E.S., E-MYCIN, ERYTHROCIN, and ILOSONE)

DOSAGE

The usual adult oral dose is initially 500 mg of base, followed by 250 mg every 6 hours. For severe infections in adults 4 g may be given daily in divided doses. The dosage in children is based on body weight: 30–50 mg/kg body weight daily in four divided doses (double for severe infections). Though the oral forms are preferred, the intravenous route may be required. For both adults and children with severe infections, 15–20 mg/kg body weight daily (maximum dose of the lactobionate salt is 4 g daily). Continuous infusion is preferable, but administration every 6 hours is also used.

CONTRAINDICATIONS AND PRECAUTIONS

Erythromycin should not be used in patients with known hypersensitivity to the drug. Caution should be exercised in patients with impaired hepatic function and those on theophylline therapy. The safety of erythromycin during pregnancy has not been established.

ADVERSE REACTIONS

Erythromycins seldom cause serious side effects, though the estolate has been reported to cause cholestatic jaundice (more so than other forms). The main side effects associated with oral erythromycin are mild gastrointestinal disturbances (nausea, vomiting, pyrosis, diarrhea), but these occur infrequently. Sensitivity reactions occur infrequently and sensorineural hearing loss (reversible) has been associated with the use of large doses of erythromycin, but is very rare. Among 375 patients on various forms of erythromycin in the Boston Collaborative Drug Surveillance Program 40 patients had side effects as follows: gastrointestinal disturbances (mainly minor, 24), sensitivity reactions (8), injection site complications (4), superinfection (3), and "other" (1).

Erythromycin can increase the effects of theophylline; the parenteral forms may be incompatible with solutions of vitamin B complex, ascorbic acid, cephalothin, tetracycline, colistin, chloramphenicol, heparin, metaraminol, and phenytoin.

LITERATURE

Lacey, RW: Postgrad Med J 53:195, 1977 (new look at erythromycin); Medical Letter, *Handbook of Antimicrobial Therapy,* rev ed 1980; Nicholas, P: NY State J Med 77:2088 and 2243, 1977 (clinical pharmacology and therapeutic uses); Olmstead, CB: Cutis:24, 414 and 422, 1979 (dermatologic use); Sanford, JP: N Engl J Med 300:654, 1979 (Legionnaire's disease); Symposium (on erythromycin); Scott Med J 22(Suppl 1):349, 1977.

ESIDRIX® (Ciba)
Hydrochlorothiazide

1981:120
1980:104
1979: 99

Hydrochlorothiazide is a diuretic and antihypertensive. Its diuretic action is due to its effect on the renal tubular mechanism of electrolyte reabsorption. The excretion of sodium and chloride occurs in approximately equal amounts and is often accompanied by a loss of potassium and bicarbonate. The mechanism of the antihypertensive action of the thiazides is unknown. Initially cardiac output falls and blood volume is diminished. With chronic therapy the cardiac output returns to normal and the peripheral vascular resistance falls.

INDICATIONS

Hydrochlorothiazide is used to treat hypertension, either alone or in combination. It is also used to treat edema associated with congestive heart failure, hepatic cirrhosis, and corticosteroid and estrogen therapy.

PREPARATIONS

Tablets: 25, 50, and 100 mg.

DOSAGE

To treat hypertension in adults, the usual starting dose is 75 mg daily as a single dose. After a week the dosage may be adjusted downward to 25 mg/day or upward to 100 mg/day. To produce diuresis in adults the initial dose range is 25–200 mg daily for several days after which 25–100 mg daily is used for maintenance. The dose for treating edema in infants and children is as follows: less than 2 years of age, 12.5–37.5 mg daily; 2–12 years of age, 37.5–100 mg daily. The dosage for infants and children may be computed based on body weight: 1 mg/lb daily.

CONTRAINDICATIONS
AND PRECAUTIONS

Anuria or hypersensitivity to this or other sulfonamide-derived drugs are contraindications. Thiazides should also not be used routinely in otherwise healthy pregnant women or nursing mothers. In patients with severe renal disease thiazides may precipitate azotemia.

ADVERSE REACTIONS Dizziness, weakness, fatigue, and leg cramps may occur. The serum potassium level frequently falls. Digitalized patients are at most risk from hypokalemia as arrhythmias can occur. Patients with cirrhosis can experience hepatic coma. The otherwise healthy ambulatory patient with hypertension usually tolerates mild hypokalemia well. Thiazides can also produce hyperglycemia and hyperuricemia. A reversible elevation in BUN can occur. Among 1058 patients on hydrochlorothiazide studied in the Boston Collaborative Drug Surveillance Program, 194 patients experienced side effects as follows: hypokalemia (82), dehydration (48), hyponatremia (16), hyperuricemia (9), asterixis (8), sensitivity reactions (9), gastrointestinal disturbances (5), hyperglycemia (3), and "other" (14).

Thiazides interact with a number of other drugs: corticosteroids, curariform agents, digitalis drugs, indomethacin, and lithium.

LITERATURE Beermann, B, Groschinsky-Grind, M: Br J Clin Pharmacol 7(6):579, 1979 (pharmacokinetics in the cardiac patient); Danielson, M, Kjellberg, J: Curr Ther Res Clin Exp 26(3):383, 1979 (hypertension—efficacy and side effects); Frohlich, ED: Drug Ther 9(2):49, 1979 (spectrum of antihypertensive theapy); Kurtzman, NA: Med Dig 25(10):5, 1979 (clinical use of diuretics); McMahon, FG: Management of Essential Hypertension, Mt Kisco, New York, Futura Publishing, 1978, Chapters 2 and 4; Medical Letter 23:45, 1981; Skoutakis, VA, et al: Clin Pharmacol Ther 25(2):249, 1979 (potassium therapy).

FASTIN® (Beecham)
Phentermine HCl

1981:177
1980:174
1979:160

Fastin is an antiobesity agent; it is a sympathomimetic amine with pharmacologic activity similar to other drugs in this class, the amphetamines, which are also used in treating obesity. Other actions include central nervous system stimulation and elevations of blood pressure. These drugs used in obesity are commonly known as anorexigenics. It has not been proved, however, that the action of these drugs in treating obesity is primarily one of appetite suppression. Other central nervous system actions or metabolic effects may be involved.

INDICATIONS	Fastin is indicated in the management of exogenous obesity as a short term adjunct in a treatment program of weight reduction based on caloric restriction.
PREPARATIONS	Capsules: 30 mg.
DOSAGE	1 capsule daily approximately 2 hours after breakfast.
CONTRAINDICATIONS AND PRECAUTIONS	Advanced arteriosclerosis, symptomatic cardiovascular disease, moderate to severe hypertension, hyperthyroidism, glaucoma, known hypersensitivity. Patients with a known history of drug abuse should not receive this drug. Further, Fastin should not be given concomitantly or within 14 days of administration of MAO inhibitors.
ADVERSE REACTIONS	Palpitations, tachycardia, and elevation of blood pressure can occur. CNS overstimulation, gastrointestinal disturbances, and allergic reactions can occur. This drug can cause a decrease in libido.
LITERATURE	Langlois, KJ, et al: Curr Ther Res 16(4):289, 1974; Moe, JF: Curr Ther Res 22(5):666, 1977.

FERROUS SULFATE

1981:158
1980:195
1979:197

Ferrous Sulfate is used in the treatment of iron deficiency anemia. In these states, the mean corpuscular volume is low, and the mean corpuscular hemoglobin concentration is low. The administration of iron is followed by an increased production of red cells in an amount proportional to the quantity of iron made available to the erythroid marrow.

INDICATIONS

Ferrous Sulfate is indicated for the treatment of iron deficient anemias.

PREPARATIONS

Capsules: 150 mg (30 mg elemental iron). Tablets: 192 and 325 mg (39 and 65 mg elemental iron, respectively). Other capsule and tablet strengths also available. Liquid preparations: available for pediatric use.

DOSAGE

For iron deficiency anemia in adults: initially 60 mg of elemental iron, increased by 30 mg increments to a maximum of 240 mg daily, given in three or four divided doses. Children, 6–12 years old: 24–120 mg elemental iron daily in three or four divided doses; 1–5 years old: 15–45 mg of elemental iron daily in three or four divided doses. Infants: 10–25 mg of elemental iron daily in three or four divided doses. For supplementation in women of child-bearing age, adolescents, and children: 18 mg of elemental iron daily is used. In pregnant and lactating women, the dosage is 25 mg of elemental iron daily. Men and postmenopausal women should receive 10 mg of elemental iron daily if supplementation is desired.

CONTRAINDICATIONS AND PRECAUTIONS

May interfere with tetracycline absorption.

111

ADVERSE REACTIONS

Adverse effects most often encountered are gastrointestinal disturbances. Among 1282 patients studied in the Boston Collaborative Drug Surveillance Program, adverse reactions were seen in 24 patients as follows: gastrointestinal disturbances (9), diarrhea (8), constipation (5), altered taste (1), and sensitivity reaction (1).

LITERATURE

Beal, RW: Drugs 2:207, 1971; Dallman, PR: J Pediatr 90:678, 1977; Savin, MA: Ration Drug Ther 11:1, 1977.

FIORINAL® (Sandoz)
Butalbital
Aspirin
Phenacetin
Caffeine

1981:46
1980:38
1979:36

Fiorinal is a combination preparation. It is used in the treatment of tension-associated headache, especially that of the head, neck, and shoulder region. Fiorinal contains the well-known analgesics aspirin and phenacetin, as well as butalbital, a barbiturate, in a concentration believed to produce minor anxiolytic and muscle relaxing effects. Caffeine, like other xanthines, constricts cerebral blood vessels and therefore may contribute to the relief of hypertensive headache. It also affects mood.

INDICATIONS

Fiorinal is indicated for the relief of the symptom complex of tension (or muscle contraction) headache.

PREPARATIONS

Tablets and capsules: 50 mg butalbial, 200 mg aspirin, 130 mg phenacetin, and 40 mg caffeine.

DOSAGE

1 or 2 tablets or capsules every 4 hours, not to exceed 6 tablets or capsules a day.

112

CONTRAINDICATIONS AND PRECAUTIONS	Not for use in patients with porphyria or in patients hypersensitive to any of the components. Not for use in the addiction-prone patient. Use cautiously in patients with peptic ulcer, coagulation abnormalities, or renal disease. The safety of this drug during pregnancy has not been fully established. Barbiturates are secreted in breast milk. The effects on infants of nursing mothers is unknown. Safety in children under 12 years of age has not been established.
ADVERSE REACTIONS	Most frequently seen are drowsiness and dizziness. Less common reactions are lightheadedness and gastrointestinal disturbances. Prolonged use of barbiturates can produce drug dependence.
LITERATURE	AMA Drug Evaluations, 4th ed. New York, AMA and Wiley, 1980, p 84; Parkhouse, J: Drugs 10:366, 1975 (on analgesics).

FIORINAL®/CODEINE (Sandoz)

1981:125
1980:108
1979:108

Butalbital
Aspirin
Caffeine
Phenacetin
Codeine phosphate

The combination of butalbital, aspirin, phenacetin and caffeine (see FIORINAL) is analgesic, anxiolytic, and muscle relaxing. The presence of codeine raises the threshold of pain and discomfort and adds an antitussive action. This preparation can be used in a variety of conditions that are painful and would otherwise require morphine.

INDICATIONS	The analgesic-sedative action of Fiorinal complements and increases the action of codeine alone. This enhanced anal-

113

gesic-sedative effect is indicated in the treatment of more severe acute and short-range periods of pain and discomfort frequently seen in office practice and in medical and surgical aftercare. The analgesic-antitussive-antipyretic action of this product makes it suitable for use in patients with upper respiratory infections.

PREPARATIONS — Capsules: 50 mg butalbital, 200 mg aspirin, 130 mg phenacetin, 40 mg caffeine, and codeine phosphate in three amounts (7.5 15 and 30 mg) for Fiorinal with codeine capsules (No. 1, No. 2, and No. 3, respectively).

DOSAGE — The usual adult dosage is 1 or 2 capsules repeated if necessary, up to 6 per day.

CONTRAINDICATIONS AND PRECAUTIONS — Should not be used in patients with known hypersensitivity to any of the components. (See also FIORINAL) Due to the barbiturate and narcotic components this drug may be habit forming and result in psychic and physical dependence and tolerance. Abrupt termination of the drug may result in withdrawal symptoms.

ADVERSE REACTIONS — Nausea, vomiting, constipation, dizziness, skin rash, drowsiness, and miosis. Note: codeine may be habit forming.

LITERATURE — See Fiorinal; also the following review on codeine: Eddy, NB, et al: Bull WHO 38:673, 1968.

FLAGYL® (Searle)
Metronidazole

1981:103
1980:103
1979:124

Metronidazole possesses direct trichomonacidal and amebacidal activity against *Trichomonas vaginalis* and *Entamoeba histolytica*, and is effective in a variety of anaerobic bacterial infection.

INDICATIONS	Symptomatic Trichomoniasis in males and females when the presence of the trichomonad has been confirmed by wet smears and/or cultures; asymptomatic trichomoniasis in females when the organism is associated with endocervicitis, cervicitis, or cervical erosion. Metronidazole also kills *Giardia lamblia* and is the agent of choice in several types of amebiasis. Flagyl has been used to treat antibiotic associated colitis (Pashby et al, 1979). Metronidazole is also effective in several anaerobic infections including intra-abdominal and pelvic infections, bone and joint infections, septic arthritis and endocarditis, meningitis and brain abscess and skin and skin structure infections caused by several Bacteroides species.
PREPARATIONS	Tablets: 250 mg and 500 mg. (The IV forms are in single dose vials containing 500 mg.)
DOSAGE	Trichomoniasis: 2 g in a 1 day treatment regimen, either as a single dose or four divided doses. An alternate course is 250 mg three times daily for 7 days. Amebiosis: In adults with acute amebic dysentery, 750 mg three times a day for 5–10 days; for amebic liver abscess; 500 or 750 mg three times a day for 5–10 days. The dose in children is based on body weight: 35–50 mg/kg in a 24 hour period given in three divided doses daily for 10 days. For anaerobic infections the IV form is used initially: 15 mg/kg infused over one hour, then followed every six hours by an infusion of 7.5 mg/kg (over one hour). When the patient is well enough oral administration of 7.5 mg/kg every six hours can be substituted. The duration of therapy is 7–10 days. (Patients with severe hepatic disease generally need lower doses

115

because of their slow rate of metabolism of the drug.)

CONTRAINDICATIONS AND PRECAUTIONS

Not to be used in patients with history of blood dyscrasia, as well as in patients with active organic disease of the central nervous system and those with history of hypersensitivity to metronidazole. This drug should not be used in the first trimester of pregnancy. Flagyl has been shown to be tumorigenic in rodents and thus should be used during the second and third trimesters of pregnancy for trichomoniasis only if other therapy has failed. Flagyl may potentiate the anticoagulant effect of coumarin and warfarin resulting in prolongation of prothrombin time. Alcohol should not be consumed during Flagyl therapy due to the possibility of nausea, cramps, vomiting, and headache.

ADVERSE REACTIONS

Most common are gastrointestinal disturbances. A metallic, sharp unpleasant taste is not unusual. Furry tongue, glossitis, and stomatitis have occurred. A moderate reversible leukopenia occurs occasionally. CNS disturbances have occurred; also mild erythematous eruptions, numbness of extremities, urticaria, flushing, nasal congestion, dryness, pruritis, dysuria, and pelvic pressure have been reported. Other adverse reactions are very rare. The urine may become darkened. Metronidazole can increase the anticoagulant effect of oral anticoagulants.

LITERATURE

Pashby, NL: Br Med J 1:1605, 1979; Rollo, IM: In The Pharmacological Basis of Therapeutics, 6th ed (Gilman, AG, Goodman, LS, Gilman, A, eds). New York, Macmillan, 1980, pp 1063, 1075–1077. For a review of use in anaerobic infections, see Medical Letter 23:13, 1981.

FLEXERIL® (Merck Sharp & Dohme)
Cyclobenzaprine HCl

1981:109
1980:134
1979:165

Flexeril relieves skeletal muscle spasm of local origin without interfering with muscle function. Its action appears to be on the brainstem. It is ineffective in muscle spasm due to central nervous system disease.

INDICATIONS	Flexeril is indicated as an adjunct to rest and physical therapy for the relief of muscle spasm associated with acute painful musculoskeletal conditions.
PREPARATIONS	Tablets: 10 mg.
DOSAGE	The dosage range of Flexeril is 20–40 mg daily in divided doses. (Not to exceed 60 mg/day.)
CONTRAINDICATIONS AND PRECAUTIONS	Flexeril should not be administered to patients with hyperthyroidism, or who are in an acute phase of recovery from myocardial infarction, have arrhythmias, heart block, conduction disturbances, or congestive heart failure. This drug should also not be used in patients known to be hypersensitive to cyclobenzaprine. Flexeril should not be used for periods of longer than 2 to 3 weeks, or with MAO inhibitors. Because of its atropine-like action, Flexeril should be used cautiously in patients with a history of urinary retention, angle-closure glaucoma, increased intraocular pressure, and in patients taking anticholinergics. Flexeril is similar in

117

structure to the tricyclic antidepressants and thus may block the antihypertensive action of guanethidine and similar compounds, and may produce arrhythmias, sinus tachycardia, and prolongation of conduction time which may lead to myocardial infarction and stoke. The safety of Flexeril in pregnancy has not been established. Flexeril is probably secreted in breast milk and thus should not be administered to the nursing mother.

ADVERSE REACTIONS

Most frequently seen are drowsiness (40%), dry mouth (28%), and dizziness (11%). Less frequently occurring are increased heart rate, weakness, fatigue, dyspepsia, nausea, paresthesia, unpleasant taste, blurred vision, and insomnia. Other reactions are rare and include sweating, myalgia, dyspnea, gastrointestinal disturbance, coated tongue, CNS effects, and allergic reactions.

LITERATURE

Basmajian, JV: Arch Phys Med Rehabil 59:58, 1978; Bercel, NA: Curr Ther Res 22:462, 1977.

GANTRISIN® (Roche)
Sulfisoxazole

1981:165
1980:139
1979:105

Gantrisin, a sulfonamide, exerts a bacteriostatic effect against a wide range of gram-positive and gram-negative microorganisms by restricting the bacterial synthesis of folic acid.

INDICATIONS

Acute, recurrent or chronic urinary infections, primarily cystitis, pyelitis, and pyclonephritis due to susceptible organisms.

118

(Oral form is preferred.) The ophthalmic solution and/or ointment is used to treat conjunctivitis, corneal ulcer, and other superficial ocular infections.

PREPARATIONS

Tablets: 0.5 g sulfisoxazole, as a pediatric suspension with each 5 ml containing approximately 0.5 g sulfisoxazole. Syrup: each 5 ml containing 0.5 g acetyl sulfisoxazole. Suspension 1 g of the long-lasting acetyl sulfisoxazole. Injectable 5 ml ampuls: each containing 2 g sulfisoxazole (each ml of the ampul contains 400 g of sulfisoxazle). Gantrisin diolamine is also available as an ophthalmic solution or ointment.

DOSAGE

Injectable forms of sulfonamides should be used only when the oral route is impractical. The usual adult dose is *initially* 2–4 g (orally). Maintenance is provided by 4–8 g daily divided into four to six doses. The usual dose for infants *over 2 months* of age and children is determined from body weight: 150 mg/kg daily. The initial dose is one half of this 24 hour maintenance dose. (Not for infants under 2 months of age.)

The injectable forms must be diluted to 5% solutions for subcutaneous and intravenous injections. The 5 ml ampul is combined with 35 ml sterile distilled water. Injectable Gantrisin is given intramuscularly without dilution. Usual dose for infants over 2 months of age, children, and adults: For maintenance 100 mg/kg daily. One half of this 24 hour dose may be given initially. (1) For subcutaneous maintenance divide the daily dose into three doses. (2) For intravenous maintenance, divide the daily dose into four doses (given slowly). (3) For intramuscular maintenance divide the daily dose into two or three doses (not more than 5 ml in any one site).

CONTRAINDICATIONS AND PRECAUTIONS

This drug should not be used in patients known to be sensitive to the sulfonamides, or in infants of less than 2 months (except in the treatment of congenital toxoplasmosis as an adjunct therapy with pyrimethamine), or in pregnancy at term and during the nursing period. Gantrisin ophthalmic preparations should not be used in patients known to be hypersensitive to sulfonamides, and are incompatible with silver preparations and may retard corneal healing. Sulfonamides should be administered with caution to patients with renal or hepatic impairment, or with severe bronchial asthma or with glucose-6-phosphate dehydrogenase deficiency. Liquid intake must be maintained due to the possibility of crystalluria and stone formation. The safe use of sulfonamides in pregnancy has not been established, but a significant increase in the formation of cleft palate and other bony abnormalities has been reported, and thus this drug should not be used in pregnancy.

ADVERSE REACTIONS

Gastrointestinal disturbances and sensitivity reactions are the most common. Blood dyscrasias and CNS reactions may occur. Toxic nephrosis, periarteritis nodosa, and L.E. phenomena have occurred. Among 427 patients studied in the Boston Collaborative Drug Surveillance Program, 20 experienced adverse effects as follows: gastrointestinal disturbances (9), sensitivity reactions (7), vasculitis (1), rise in BUN (2), and "other" (1).

Sulfonamides interact with oral anticoagulants, hypoglycemics, thiopental sodium, and other drugs which compete for the same protein binding site to which the sulfonamide binds.

LITERATURE   Mandell, GL, Sande, MA: In The Pharma-cological Basis of Therapeutics, 6th ed. (Gilman, AG, Goodman, LS, Gilman, A, eds). New York, Macmillan, 1980, p 1110; Medical Letter 23:69, 1981.

GYNE—LOTRIMIN® (Schering)
Clotrimazole

1981:156
1980:168
1979:191

Clotrimazole, an antibiotic vaginal preparation, has a broad spectrum antifungal action that inhibits the growth of pathogenic yeasts.

INDICATIONS

Gyne-Lotrimin vaginal cream is indicated for the local treatment of patients with vulvovaginal candidiasis.

PREPARATIONS

Vaginal cream: 1% with approximately 50 mg clotrimazole. Tablets: 100 mg of clotrimazole.

DOSAGE

Cream: 1 applicatorful a day for 7–14 consecutive days. Tablets: 1 tablet intravaginally (at bedtime) for 7 consecutive days.

CONTRAINDICATIONS AND PRECAUTIONS

These preparations are not to be used in patients who have shown hypersensitivity in the past. There is no information concerning the safety of this product in the first trimester of pregnancy, but no ill effects are associated with its use in the second and third trimesters.

ADVERSE REACTIONS

Adverse reactions include vaginal burning, erythema, irritation, lower abdominal cramps, and burning or irritation in the sexual partner. The incidence of adverse

121

reactions is somewhat lower with the cream (0.5%) than for the tablets (1.6%).

LITERATURE   Ipp, MM, et al: Am J Dis Child 131:305, 1977; Sawyer, PR, et al: Drugs 9:424, 1975.

HALDOL® (McNeil)
Haloperidol

1981: 99
1980:119
1979:137

Haloperidol is one of the major tranquilizers. Its precise mechanism of action has not been clearly established.

INDICATIONS

Haldol is indicated for use in the management of the symptoms of psychotic disorders. It is indicated for the control of tics, and vocal utterances of the Gilles de la Tourette's syndrome in children and adults. Haloperidol is also effective for the treatment of severe behavioral problems in children of combative explosive hyperexcitability. It is also effective in the short-term treatment of hyperactive children who show excessive motor activity with accompanying conduct disorders.

PREPARATIONS

Tablets: 0.5, 1, 2, 5, 10 and 20 mg. Concentate: 2 mg/ml. Injection ampuls: 1 ml ampule, 10 ml multiple dose vial and 1 ml disposable syringe, each containing 5 mg/ml.

DOSAGE

The initial (and maintenance) dosage depends on the patients age, severity of illness, previous response to other neuroleptic drugs, and any concomitant medication or disease state. The following ranges are recommended: *Oral* administration for moderate symptomatology: 0.5–2.0 mg two or three times a day; for severe symptomatology: 3.0–5.0 mg two or three times a day. Upon achieving a satisfactory therapeutic response the maintenance dosage should be gradually reduced to the lowest effective maintenance level. *Intramuscular* administration is used for prompt control of the acutely agitated patient with moderately severe to very severe symptoms. The dosage range via this route is 2–5 mg and repeated if needed as often as every hour.

CONTRAINDICATIONS AND PRECAUTIONS

This drug should not be administered to patients who have a severely depressed central nervous system due to alcohol or other depressants, are comatose, are severely depressed, or have Parkinson's disease. Haldol should also be avoided in individuals who are hypersensitive to this drug. Since experience does not exclude the possibility of fetal damage due to haloperidol, this drug should be used in pregnancy only when the benefits clearly justify a potential risk to the fetus. Furthermore, infants should not be nursed while the drug is being used. Concomitant treatment with lithium should be avoided, due to the possibility of encephalopathic syndromes which may be followed by irreversible brain damage. Treatment should be discontinued if signs of bronchopneumonia appear. Because of mental impairment by this drug, ambulatory patients should be warned of the hazards of tasks requiring alertness (such as driving a car). Alcohol should be avoided while Haldol is being used due to the possibility of additive effects. Haldol should be administered cautiously to patients with severe cardiovascular disorders (due to the possibility of transient hypotension and the precipitation of anginal pain). Haldol changes the threshold to seizure and thus should be avoided in patients who are receiving anticonvulsant medication. In addition, Haldol should be avoided in patients with known history of allergy to drugs, who are receiving anticoagulants, and only with great caution in patients receiving concomitant therapy for Parkinsonism. Haldol used to control mania may result in severe mood swings toward depression. Severe neurotoxicity (rigidity, inability to walk or talk) may occur in patients with thyrotoxicosis who are also receiving antipsychotic medication including Haldol.

ADVERSE REACTIONS

Extrapyramidal reactions have been reported frequently during the first few days of treatment. Persistent dyskinesias may occur, but have been reported rarely. Other CNS reactions may occur and autonomic effects including tachycardia and hypotension may occur, although less often than with phenothiazines. Hematologic, hepatic, and dermatologic reactions occur rarely and are usually mild. Barbiturates and phenytoin decrease haloperidol effects. Its toxicity may be increased by lithium and methyldopa.

LITERATURE

Ayd, FJ, Jr: J Clin Psychiatry 39(11):807, 1978 (a report on 20 years of clinical experience with haloperidol).

HYDERGINE® (Sandoz)
Dihydroergocornine mesylate
Dihydroergocristine mesylate
Dihydroergocryptine mesylate

1981:157
1980:160
1979:170

Hydergine is a mixture of dihydrogenated ergot alkaloids. It has mental effects whose mechanisms of action have not been clearly established, but there is some evidence for its possible efficacy in treating senile dementias. There is no conclusive evidence that the drug has any significant effect in the treatment of cerebral arterial sclerosis or cerebral vascular insufficiency.

INDICATIONS

Hydergine tablets and sublingual tablets are indicated for the treatment of selected symptoms in elderly patients. Short-term clinical studies have shown modest improvements in levels of performance of self-care, and such symptoms as depression, confusion, unsociability, and dizziness.

PREPARATIONS

Tablets: 1 mg (oral use) and 1 and 0.5 mg (sublingual use). Each 1 mg contains dihydroergocornine mesylate 0.333 mg, dihydroergocristine mesylate 0.333 mg, and dihydroergocryptine mesylate 0.333 mg. Liquid: 1 mg/ml in bottles of 100 ml.

DOSAGE

1 mg three times daily. Alleviation of symptoms is gradual (3–4 weeks).

CONTRAINDICATIONS
AND PRECAUTIONS

Not to be used in patients who have previously shown hypersensitivity to the drug and in patients with acute or chronic psychosis.

ADVERSE REACTIONS

Sublingual irritation, gastric disturbances, and transient nausea have been reported.

LITERATURE   Bazo, AJ: J Am Geriatrics Soc 21:63, 1973;
                    Ditch, M, et al: J Am Geriatrics Soc
                    19:208, 1971; Einspruch, BC: Dis Nerv
                    Syst 37:439, 1976; Gaitz, CM, et al: Arch
                    Gen Psychiatry 34:839, 1977.

HYDRALAZINE HCl

1981:183
1980: —
1979: —

Hydralazine lowers blood pressure by means of a direct relaxing action on vascular smooth muscle.

INDICATIONS   Hydralazine is indicated for the treatment
                     of essential hypertension either alone or
                     as an adjunct to other therapy.

PREPARATIONS   Tablets: 10, 25, 50, and 100 mg. Injecta-
                     ble form (used only when the oral route
                     cannot be used): 1 ml ampuls each con-
                     taining 20 mg hydralazine hydrochloride
                     and preservatives in water.

DOSAGE   When initiating therapy in adults with hy-
                     dralazine as the sole therapeutic agent the
                     dose is 10 mg four times a day for 2–4
                     days then followed by 25 mg four times
                     a day for the rest of the week. For the
                     second and subsequent weeks the dosage
                     may be increased to 50 mg four times
                     daily. The incidence of toxic reactions
                     may be higher with larger doses of hydral-
                     azine. In these cases a lower dose of hy-
                     dralazine may be combined with a thiazide
                     or other antihypertensive drug. When
                     used parenterally (only when the oral
                     route is impossible or in emergencies) the
                     usual dose is 20–40 mg intravenously or
                     intramuscularly. A fall in blood pressure

may occur in 10–80 minutes after injection.

CONTRAINDICATIONS
AND PRECAUTIONS

Hydralazine is contraindicated in patients with coronary artery disease and with mitral valvular rheumatic heart disease. It should also not be used in patients with previous demonstration of hypersensitivity to the drug or in pregnant women.

ADVERSE REACTIONS

In some patients hydralazine may produce a syndrome that resembles systemic lupus erythematosus. Common side effects include headache, palpitations, anorexia, nausea, vomiting, diarrhea, tachycardia, and angina pectoris. The Boston Collaborative Drug Surveillance Program (BCDSP) studied 223 patients on hydralazine and reported hypotension as the most frequent adverse reaction (22 patients) followed by headache (8), gastrointestinal disturbances (4), tachycardia or palpitations (3), rise in BUN (2), and "other" (2). BCDSP reported two severe adverse reactions in patients receiving parenteral hydralazine because of severe hypertension.

Less frequent adverse reactions are nasal congestion, flushing, lacrimation, conjunctivitis, peripheral neuritis, edema, dizziness, tremors, muscle cramps, and psychotic reactions. Constipation and difficulty in micturition have also been reported as have dyspnea, paralytic ileus, lymphadenopathy, splenomegaly, and blood dyscrasias. Paradoxical pressor response has also been reported.

MAO inhibitors should be used cautiously in patients receiving hydralazine. When other powerful antihypertensive drugs are used with hydralazine given parenterally the patient should be watched for any excessive fall in blood pressure.

127

LITERATURE   Hollander, W: Clin Ther 2(Suppl A):11,
1979; McMahon, FG: Management of Essential Hypertension, Futura Publishing,
Mount Kisco, New York, 1978, pp 209–
249. *For information and references on the use
of hydralazine and other vasodilators in the
treatment of congestive heart failure,* see Fitch-
ett, DH, et al: Am J Cardiol 44(2):303,
1979; Medical Letter 20:89, 1978.

HYDROCHLOROTHIAZIDE

1981:17
1980:29
1979:41

Hydrochlorothiazide is a diuretic and antihypertensive. Its diuretic
action is due to its effect on the renal tubular mechanism of electrolyte reabsorption. The excretion of sodium and chloride occurs in
approximately equal amounts and is often accompanied by a loss
of potassium and bicarbonate. The mechanism of the antihypertensive action of the thiazides is unknown. Initially cardiac output falls
and blood volume is diminished. With chronic therapy the cardiac
output returns to normal and the peripheral vascular resistance falls.

INDICATIONS   Hydrochlorothiazide is used to treat hypertension, either alone or in combina-
tion. It is also useful in treating edema
that is associated with congestive heart
failure, hepatic cirrhosis, and corticosteroid and estrogen therapy.

PREPARATIONS   (Several manufacturers) Tablets: 25, 50,
and 100 mg. (See ESIDRIX, HYDRODI-
URIL)

DOSAGE   To treat hypertension in adults, the usual
starting dose is 75 mg daily as a single
dose. After a week the dosage may be adjusted downward to 25 mg/day or upward
to 100 mg/day. To produce diuresis in
adults the initial dose range is 25–200 mg

128

daily for several days after which 25–100 mg daily is used for maintenance. The dose for treating edema in infants and children is as follows: less than 2 years of age, 12.5–37.5 mg daily; between 2 and 12 years of age, 37.5–100 mg daily. The dosage for infants and children may be computed based on body weight: 1 mg/lb daily.

CONTRAINDICATIONS AND PRECAUTIONS

Anuria or hypersensitivity to this or other sulfonamide-derived drugs are contraindications. Thiazides should also not be used routinely in otherwise healthy pregnant women or nursing mothers. In patients with severe renal disease thiazides may precipitate azotemia.

ADVERSE REACTIONS

Dizziness, weakness, fatigue, and leg cramps may occur. The serum potassium level frequently falls. Digitalized patients are at most risk from hypokalemia as arrhythmias can occur. Patients with cirrhosis can experience hepatic coma. The otherwise healthy ambulatory patient with hypertension usually tolerates mild hypokalemia well. Thiazides can also produce hyperglycemia and hyperuricemia. A reversible elevation in BUN can occur. Among 1058 patients on hydrochlorothiazide studied in the Boston Collaborative Drug Surveillance Program, 194 patients experienced side effects as follows: hypokalemia (82), dehydration (48), hyponatremia (16), hyperuricemia (9), asterixis (8), sensitivity reactions (9), gastrointestinal disturbances (5), hyperglycemia (3), and "other" (14).

Thiazides interact with a number of other drugs: corticosteroids, curariform agents, digitalis drugs, indomethacin, and lithium.

129

LITERATURE   Beermann, B, Groschinsky-Grind, M: Br
              J Clin Pharmacol 7(6):579, 1979 (pharma-
              cokinetics in the cardiac patient); Daniel-
              son, M, Kjellberg, J: Curr Ther Res Clin
              Exp 26(3):383, 1979 (hypertension—effi-
              cacy and side effects); Frohlich, ED: Drug
              Ther 9(2):49, 1979 (spectrum of antihy-
              pertensive therapy); Kurtzman, NA: Med
              Dig 25(10):5, 1979 (clinical use of diuret-
              ics); McMahon, FG: Management of Es-
              sential Hypertension. Mount Kisco, New
              York, Futura Publishing, 1978, Chapters
              2 and 4; Medical Letter 23:45, 1981;
              Skoutakis, VA, et al: Clin Pharamacol Ther
              25(2):249, 1979 (potassium therapy).

HYDROCORTISONE (Dermatologic)   1981:153
                                          1980:189
                                          1979: —

Topical steroids are primarily effective because of their anti-inflammatory, antipruritic, and vasoconstrictive action.

INDICATIONS   The agents are used to relieve the inflam-
                      matory manifestations of corticosteroid-
                      responsive dermatoses.

PREPARATIONS   Creams: 0.125–1.0%. Lotions: 0.125–
                      0.25%. Ointments: 1–2.5%. Gels: 1%.
                      Aerosols: 0.5%.

DOSAGE   Application is to the affected areas three
                      or four times daily.

CONTRAINDICATIONS   Patients with known hypersensitivity
AND PRECAUTIONS   should not use these preparations.

ADVERSE REACTIONS   Burning, itching, irritation, dryness, and
                      folliculitis can occur. Pigmentation, acne-
                      form eruptions, maceration of the skin,

130

skin atrophy, striae, and miliaria can develop.

LITERATURE   Sneddon, IB: Drugs 11:193, 1976; Stoughton, RB: In Recent Advances in Dermatopharmacology (Frost, P, et al, eds). New York, Spectrum, 1978, pp 105–112.

HYDRODIURIL® (Merck Sharp & Dohme)
Hydrochlorothiazide

1981:22
1980:20
1979:16

Hydrochlorothiazide is a diuretic and antihypertensive. Its diuretic action is due to its effect on the renal tubular mechanism of electrolyte reabsorption. The excretion of sodium and chloride occurs in approximately equal amounts and is often accompanied by a loss of potassium and bicarbonate. The mechanism of the antihypertensive action of the thiazides is unknown. Initially cardiac output falls and blood volume is diminished. With chronic therapy the cardiac output returns to normal and the peripheral vascular resistance falls.

INDICATIONS   Hydrochlorothiazide is used to treat hypertension, either alone or in combination. It is also useful in treating edema that is associated with congestive heart failure, hepatic cirrhosis, and corticosteroid and estrogen therapy.

PREPARATIONS   Tablets: 25, 50, and 100 mg.

DOSAGE   To treat hypertension in adults, the usual starting dose is 75 mg daily as a single dose. After a week the dosage may be adjusted downward to 25 mg/day or upward to 100 mg/day. To produce diuresis in adults the initial dose range is 25–200 mg daily for several days after which 25–100 mg daily is used for maintenance. The

131

dose for treating edema in infants and children is as follows: less than 2 years of age, 12.5–37.5 mg daily; 2–12 years of age, 37.5–100 mg daily. The dosage for infants and children may be computed based on body weight; 1 mg/lb daily.

CONTRAINDICATIONS AND PRECAUTIONS

Anuria or hypersensitivity to this or other sulfonamide-derived drugs are contraindications. Thiazides should also not be used routinely in otherwise healthy pregnant women or nursing mothers. In patients with severe renal disease thiazides may precipitate azotemia.

ADVERSE REACTIONS

Dizziness, weakness, fatigue, and leg cramps may occur. The serum potassium level frequently falls. Digitalized patients are at more risk from hypokalemia as arrhythmias can occur. Patients with cirrhosis can experience hepatic coma. The otherwise healthy ambulatory patient with hypertension usually tolerates mild hypokalemia well. Thiazides can also produce hyperglycemia and hyperuricemia. A reversible elevation in BUN can occur. Among 1058 patients on hydrochlorothiazide studied in the Boston Collaborative Drug Surveillance Program, 194 patients experienced side effects as follows: hypokalemia (82), dehydration (48), hyponatremia (16), hyperuricemia (9), asterixis (8), sensitivity reactions (9), gastrointestinal disturbances (5), hyperglycemia (3), and "other" (14).

Thiazides interact with a number of other drugs: corticosteroids, curariform agents, digitalis drugs, indomethacin, and lithium.

LITERATURE

Beermann, B, Groschinsky-Grind, M: Br J Clin Pharmacol 7(6):579, 1979 (pharmacokinetics in the cardiac patient); Danielson, M, Kjellberg, J: Curr Ther Res Clin Exp 26(3):383, 1979 (hypertension—efficacy and side effects); Frohlich, ED: Drug Ther 9(2):49, 1979 (spectrum of antihypertensive therapy); Kurtzman, NA: Med Dig 25(10):5, 1979 (clinical use of diuretics); McMahon, FG: Management of Essential Hypertension, Mt. Kisco, New York, Futura Publishing, 1978, Chapters 2 and 4; Medical Letter 23:45, 1981; Skoutakis, VA, et al: Clin Pharmacol Ther 25(2):249, 1979 (potassium therapy).

HYDROPRES® (Merck Sharp & Dohme)
Hydrochlorothiazide
Reserpine

1981:119
1980:126
1979:111

The actions of Hydropres are those of its constituent agents. Hydrochlorothiazide is a diuretic and antihypertensive (See HYDROCHLOROTHIAZIDE). Reserpine is an antihypertensive with bradycardic action and tranquilizing properties that are consequences of its property of depleting catecholamines from central and peripheral sites.

INDICATIONS	Hydropres is indicated in the treatment of hypertension.
PREPARATIONS	Hydropres-25 tablets: 25 mg hydrochlorothiazide and 0.125 mg reserpine; Hydropres-50 tablets: 50 mg hydrochlorothiazide and 0.125 mg reserpine.
DOSAGE	The usual adult dosage of Hydropres-25 is 1 or 2 tablets once or twice a day. When Hydropres-50 is used the usual adult dosage is 1 tablet once or twice a day. Adjustment of dosage is based on patient response.

Hydrochlorothiazide is contraindicated in anuria. Sensitivity to hydrochlorothiazide, other sulfonamide-derived drugs, or reserpine precludes the use of this preparation. Electroshock therapy is not to be employed while reserpine is being given due to fatal reactions associated with minimal electroshock dosage; 7 days should be allowed following reserpine treatment before the use of electroshock. Active peptic ulcer, ulcerative colitis, and active mental depression (particularly with suicidal tendencies) are contraindications to reserpine. This preparation should not be administered to patients with renal or hepatic impairment, and Hydropres may add to the effects of other antihypertensive agents. Sensitivity may occur in patients with or without history of bronchial asthma, and systemic lupus erythematosus may result. Lithium should not be given with this preparation. This preparation should be discontinued with any signs of mental depression. The following electrolyte imbalances may occur: hyponatremia, hypochloremic alkalosis, hypokalemia (resulting in increased sensitivity to the heart to digitalis), and hyperuricemia (resulting in the possibility of the precipitation of gout). Insulin requirements may be altered in diabetics, and latent diabetes mellitus may be precipitated. There may be an increased sensitvity to tubocurarine, and the antihypertensive effects of this preparation may be increased in the postsympathectomy patient. In addition, there is a decreased arterial responsiveness to norepinephrine. Reserpine may increase gastric secretion and motility, and should not be used in patients with peptic ulcer, ulcerative colitis, or other gastrointestinal disorders. In addition, this compound may precipitate gallstones or bronchial asthma in susceptible persons, and cause hypotension (including orthostatic hypotension). Caution should be exercised in pregnancy since reserpine crosses the placental barrier, and thiazides and reserpine appear in breast milk, thus indicating that unless use of the drug is deemed essential it should not be used by nursing mothers.

ADVERSE REACTIONS

The adverse reactions of Hydropres are those associated with each of its components (see HYDROCHLOROTHIAZIDE). Reserpine affects the central nervous system, producing in some cases excessive sedation, mental depression, nightmares, headache, dizziness, and syncope. It also may produce other CNS effects. The actions of reserpine on the cardiovascular system include bradycardia, angina pectoris, arrhythmias, fluid retention, and congestive failure. Gastrointestinal, hematologic, allergic, and other reactions may also occur. Among 213 patients receiving reserpine drugs in the Boston Collaborative Drug Surveillance Program, approximately 10% experienced adverse reactions, the most frequent being hypotension, drowsiness, headache or vertigo, and depression.

Reserpine interacts with general anesthetics and with sympathomimetic amines.

LITERATURE

Duhme, DW, et al: Am J Hosp Pharm 32(5):508, 1975; Smith, WM: Hosp Formulary Manag 11(1):25, 1976. For a thorough discussion of reserpine, see McMahon, FG: Management of Essential Hypertension. Mount Kisco, New York, Futura Publishing, 1978, Chapter 12; Medical Letter 23:45, 1981.

HYGROTON® (USV)
Chlorthalidone

1981:27
1980:30
1979:27

Hygroton, an oral antihypertensive-diuretic, has a prolonged action; that is, 48–72 hours. The diuretic effect occurs within 2 hours of an oral dose and continues up to 72 hours. It produces an effective diuresis with increased excretion of sodium and chloride.

INDICATIONS — Hygroton is indicated in the management of hypertension. It is sometimes used alone or sometimes used in combination with other antihypertensive drugs. It is also used as adjunctive therapy to treat edema due to various conditions.

PREPARATIONS — Tablets: 25, 50, and 100 mg.

DOSAGE — Hypertension: Therapy should be initiated with a single daily dose of 25 or 50 mg (not above 100 mg). The maintenance dose may be lowered based on patient responses. Edema: Initiation dose range in adults is 50–100 mg daily (not above 200 mg). Maintenance doses may be lowered based on patient response.

CONTRAINDICATIONS AND PRECAUTIONS — Chlorthalidone is not to be used in anuria, or when patients are known to be hypersensitive to chlorthalidone or other sulfonamide-derived drugs. Caution should be exercised in patients with severe renal disease and in those with impaired hepatic function. Potentiation or additive effects may result from combined therapy with other antihypertensive drugs. Use cautiously in asthmatics and in pregnant women and nursing mothers.

ADVERSE REACTIONS — Gastrointestinal disturbances, CNS reactions (dizziness, vertigo, paresthesias,

136

headache, xanthopsia), hematologic reactions, and hypersensitivity dermatologic reactions may occur. Orthostatic hypotension may occur. Other reported untoward effects are hypokalemia, hyperglycemia, glycosuria, hyperuricemia, muscle spasm, weakness, restlessness, and impotence.

LITERATURE

Finnerty, FA: Angiology 27(12):738, 1976; Kakaviatos, N, Finnerty, FA: Am J Cardiol 10(4):570, 1962; Medical Letter 23:45, 1981.

ILOSONE® (Dista)
Erythromycin estolate

1981:98
1980:84
1979:43

Erythromycin, from the macrolide group of antibiotics, inhibits bacterial protein synthesis. It is widely used as an alternate to penicillin and is one of the safest antibiotics currently in use. Besides its use as an alternate to penicillin, erythromycin is the recommended drug in many disease states. It diffuses readily into most body fluids, but only low concentrations are achieved in the spinal fluid. The oral forms are preferred though these are inactivated to varying degrees by gastric juice.

INDICATIONS

Erythromycin is effective in the treatment of infections caused by S. pyogenes, S. aureus, S. pneumoniae, M. pneumoniae, H. influenza (concomitant with a sulfonamide), Treponema pallidum and L. monocytogenes. Erythromycin is used in Legionnaire's disease, chlamydial infections, intestinal amebiases, erythrasma, and as an adjunct to antitoxin in the treatment of diphtheria. Erythromycin is also effective in

Bordetella pertussis (whooping cough) in eliminating the organism from the nasopharynx of infected individuals and may be used with injectable (lactobionate) forms as an alternate treatment of acute pelvic inflammation caused by *N. gonorrhoeae* in female patients sensitive to penicillin. Injectable penicillin G benzathine is recommended by the American Heart Association in the treatment and prevention of streptococcal pharyngitis and long-term prophylaxis of rheumatic fever. Oral penicillin G or V or erythromycin are alternates in the above conditions. Erythromycin is used by patients with a history of heart disease and who are sensitive to penicillin for short-term prophylaxis prior to dental procedures.

PREPARATIONS

Capsules: 125 and 250 mg. Granules for suspension: 125 mg in 5 ml after reconstitution. Suspension: 125 and 250 mg per 5 ml. Tablets (chewable): 125 and 250 mg. Tablets: 500 mg.

DOSAGE

Adults: 250 mg every 6 hours. Children: age, weight, and severity are important factors. Usually 30–50 mg/kg per day in divided doses.

CONTRAINDICATIONS AND PRECAUTIONS

Erythromycin should not be used in patients with known hypersensitivity to the drug. Caution should be exercised in patients with impaired hepatic function and those on theophylline therapy. The safety of erythromycin during pregnancy has not been established.

ADVERSE REACTIONS

Erythromycins seldom cause serious side effects, though the estolate has been reported to cause hepatic dysfunction and cholestatic jaundice (more so than other forms). The main side effects associated with oral erythromycin are mild gastrointestinal disturbances (nausea, vomiting, pyrosis, diarrhea), but these occur infrequently. Sensitivity reactions occur infrequently and sensorineural hearing loss (reversible) has been associated with the use of large doses of erythromycin, but is very rare. Among 375 patients on various forms of erythromycin in the Boston Collaborative Drug Surveillance Program 40 patients had side effects as follows: gastrointestinal disturbances (mainly minor, 24), sensitivity reactions (8), injection site complications (4), superinfection (3), and "other" (1).

Erythromycin can increase the effects of theophylline; the parenteral forms may be incompatible with solutions of vitamin B complex, ascorbic acid, cephalothin, tetracycline, colistin, chloramphenicol, heparin, metaraminol, and phenytoin.

LITERATURE

Lacey, RW: Postgrad Med J 53:195, 1977 (new look at erythromycin); Medical Letter 24:21, 1982 (choice of antimicrobials); Nicholas, P: NY State J Med 77:2088 and 2243, 1977 (clinical pharmacology and therapeutic uses); Olmstead, CB: Cutis 24:414 and 422, 1979 (dermatologic use); Sanford, JP: N Engl J Med 300:654, 1979 (Legionnaire's disease); Symposium (on erythromycin): Scott Med J 22 (Suppl 1):349, 1977.

IMODIUM® (Ortho)
Loperamide HCl

1981:200
1980: —
1979: —

Imodium is a synthetic antidiarrheal for oral use that acts by slowing intestinal motility and by effecting water and electrolyte movement through the bowel. It inhibits peristaltic activity by a direct effect on the circular and longitudinal muscles of the intestinal wall.

INDICATIONS	Imodium is indicated for the control and symptomatic relief of acute non-specific diarrhea and of chronic diarrhea associated with inflammatory bowel disease. Imodium is also indicated for reducing the volume of discharge from ileostomies.
PREPARATIONS	Capsules: 2 mg.
DOSAGE	For acute diarrhea: 2 capsules (4 mg) followed by one capsule (2 mg) after each unformed stool (not to exceed 16 mg daily). For treating chronic diarrhea, the initial dose is two capsules (4 mg), followed by one capsule (2 mg) after each unformed stool until diarrhea is controlled, after which the dosage should be decreased to meet individual requirements. The average daily maintenance dose is 4 to 8 mg.
CONTRAINDICATIONS AND PRECAUTIONS	Imodium is contraindicated in patients with known hypersensitivity to the drug and in patients in whom constipation must be avoided. Antiperistaltic agents should not be used in acute diarrhea associated with organisms that penetrate the intestinal mucosa such as enterovasive *E. Coli, Salmonella, and Shigella,* and in pseudomembranous colitis associated with broad-spectrum antibiotics. In acute diarrhea, if clinical symptoms do not improve

140

in 48 hours, the use of Imodium should be discontinued. Safe use of Imodium during pregnancy has not been established. It is not known whether this drug is excreted in human milk. This drug is not recommended for children under the age of 12.

ADVERSE REACTIONS   The following adverse effects were recorded during clinical trials but are difficult to distinguish from symptoms associated with the diarrheal syndrome: Abdominal pain and discomfort, constipation, drowsiness, dizziness, dry mouth, nausea and vomiting, and tiredness. Hyersensitivity reactions, including skin rash, have also been reported.

LITERATURE   Jaffe, JH et al: Clin Pharm Ther 28:812, 1980 (abuse potential); Niemegeers, CJE et al: Arzneim-Forsch (Drug Research) 24:1636, 1974 (a novel type of antidiarrheal agent); Niemegeers, CJE, McGuire, JL: Proc FASEB 36:1019, 1977 (antidiarrheal specificity of loperamide); Weintraub, HS et al: Curr Ther Res 21:867, 1977 (pharmacokinetics).

INDERAL® (Ayerst)   1981:2
Propranolol HCl   1980:2
1979:2

Inderal is a beta-adrenergic receptor-blocking drug. It is specifically competitive with beta-adrenergic receptor stimulating agents. The chronotropic, inotropic, and vasodilator responses of beta-adrenergic agents are blocked by Inderal. This drug decreases heart rate, cardiac output, and blood pressure. The mechanism of the antihypertensive effect of propranolol has not been completely determined but may be related to the decreased cardiac output, inhibition of renin release by the kidneys and reduction in central sympathetic

141

outflow. (A newer use is after myocardial infarction. See JAMA reference.)

INDICATIONS

Inderal is indicated in the management of hypertension. It is usually used in combination with other drugs, particularly a thiazide diuretic. It is also used in selected patients for the treatment of angina pectoris in patients with moderate or severe angina who do not respond to conventional methods. Inderal is also used to treat supraventricular arrhythmias such as paroxysmal atrial tachycardia, persistent sinus atrial tachycardia which is noncompensatory, tachycardia and arrhythmias due to thyrotoxicosis and persistent atrial extrasystoles, and atrial flutter and fibrillation when digitalis alone is not adequate or when it is contraindicated. Ventricular tachycardia and ventricular arrhythmias do not respond predictably to propranolol but it may be of some value. Digitalis-induced tachyarrhythmias, which persist after stopping digitalis and correcting electrolyte abnormalities, are often reversible with oral propranolol. Propranolol is also useful in the management of hypertrophic subaortic stenosis, especially for treatment of exertional or stress-induced angina, palpitations and syncope. Another use of Inderal is in the prophylaxis of common migraine headache. It is not useful once the migraine attack has already started.

PREPARATIONS

Tablets: 10, 20, 40, and 80 mg. Ampuls: 1 ml containing 1 mg of propranolol hydrochloride.

DOSAGE

The dosage range for Inderal is different for each indication and, generally, the

142

dosage must be individualized. The following are usual adult dosage ranges:

1. *Hypertension.* Initially, 80 mg daily in two divided doses, then gradually increased to 160–480 mg daily in two divided doses.

2. *Angina pectoris.* Initially 10–20 mg three or four times daily. Increase gradually to 160 mg daily. (Not to exceed 320 mg per day.) If treatment is to be discontinued reduce dosage gradually over a period of several weeks.

3. *Arrhythmias.* 10–30 mg three or four times daily.

4. *Migraines.* The initial oral dose is 80 mg daily in divided doses. The usual effective range is 160–240 mg per day.

5. *Hypertrophic subaortic stenosis.* 20–40 mg three or four times daily.

Note 1. Information on the use of this drug in infants and children is inadequate at present.

Note 2. Intravenous administration is used only for life threatening arrhythmias. The rate should not exceed 1 mg per minute and the usual range is 1–3 mg administered under careful monitoring.

CONTRAINDICATIONS AND PRECAUTIONS

Inderal should not be used in patients with bronchial asthma, allergic rhinitis (during the pollen season), sinus bradycardia and greater than first degree block, cardiogenic shock, right ventricular failure secondary to pulmonary hypertension, congestive heart failure (unless heart failure is secondary to a tachyarrhythmia which is treatable with Inderal), in combination with adrenergic-augmenting psychotropic drugs (including monoamine oxidase inhibitors), and during the 2 week withdrawal from such drugs. Caution should be used in cardiac failure (Inderal may precipitate cardiac failure in patients without a history of cardiac failure), or in patients with thyrotoxicosis or with Wolff-Parkinson-White syndrome. Care must also be exercised in patients under anesthesia and those undergoing major surgery (due to impairment of cardiac reflexes). Inderal should also be used cautiously in patients with nonallergic bronchospasm (eg, chronic emphysema) and in diabetes and patients subject to hypoglycemia. The concomitant use of catecholamine depleting drugs such as reserpine should be closely monitored. The safe use of Inderal in pregnancy has not been established.

ADVERSE REACTIONS

Cardiovascular reactions may occur: bradycardia, conduction disturbances, and hypotension are the most common. CNS reactions including lightheadedness, mental depression, weakness, and fatigue can occur. Gastrointestinal disturbances, bronchospasm, hematologic, and allergic reactions can also occur. Among 487 patients on propranolol studied in the Boston Collaborative Drug Surveillance Program, 42 patients experienced adverse reactions as follows: bradycardia or conduction disturbances (11), hypotension (10), neuropsychiatric reactions (5), congestive heart failure or fluid retention (4), sensitivity reactions (3), pulmonary edema (2), shock (2), azotemia (2), bronchospasms (2), gastrointestinal disturbances (1).

Propranolol interacts with a number of drugs: general anesthetics, barbiturates, chlorpromazine, clonidine, furosemide, oral hypoglycemics, indomethacin, lidocaine, sympathomimetic amines and protriptyline (see Medical Letter reference).

144

LITERATURE   Elliott, WC, Stone, JM: Prog Cardiovasc Dis 12:83, 1969 (angina pectoris); Gibson, D, Sowton, E: Prog Cardiovasc Dis 12:16, 1969 (arrhythmias); Malcolm, J: Acta Cardiol Suppl 15:307, 1972, (hyperthyroidism); Medical Letter 23(5):17, 1981 (interactions); Medical Letter 23:45, 1981 (drugs for hypertension); Veterans Administration Cooperative Study Group, JAMA 237(21):2303, 1977 (on propranolol in hypertension); Friedman, LM: JAMA 247:1707, 1982; Weber, RG, Reinmuth, OM: Neurology 22:366, 1972 (migraine). See also: Inderal, A Compendium of Abstracts. Ayerst Laboratories, 1979.

INDOCIN® (Merck Sharp & Dohme)
Indomethacin

1981:25
1980:24
1979:21

Indocin is a nonsteroidal drug with anti-inflammatory, anti-pyretic, and analgesic properties. Its mode of action is not known, but it is known that indomethacin is a potent inhibitor of prostaglandin synthesis in vitro. Indocin has been shown to be effective as an anti-inflammatory agent for long-term use in rheumatoid arthritis, ankylosing spondylitis, and osteoarthritis. It affords relief of symptoms, but does not alter the progressive course of the underlying disease.

INDICATIONS   Moderate to severe rheumatoid arthritis including acute flares in chronic disease, moderate to severe ankylosing spondylitis, moderate to severe osteoarthritis of the large joints, and in acute gouty arthritis. Indocin is not a simple analgesic; hence it should be used only in those conditions for which it is specifically indicated.

145

PREPARATIONS	Capsules: 25 and 50 mg.

DOSAGE The smallest dosage that is effective for the patient should be used in order to minimize adverse effects. The drug should always be taken with food, immediately after meals or with antacids to reduce gastric distress. The initial suggested dosage for all indications, except acute gouty arthritis, is 25 mg two or three times a day. If tolerated the daily dosage may be increased by 25 or 50 mg (not to exceed a total daily dose of 200 mg). For acute gouty arthritis the suggested dosage is 50 mg three times a day until the pain is tolerable, then the dose should be rapidly reduced.

CONTRAINDICATIONS AND PRECAUTIONS Indocin should not be used in patients who are sensitive to indomethacin or who have nasal polyps associated with angioedema or bronchospastic reaction to aspirin or other nonsteroidal anti-inflammatory drugs. Greater caution must be exercised in prescribing this compound to the aged or the young (Indocin should ordinarily not be given to children under the age of 14 years). Gastrointestinal effects associated with Indocin are single or multiple ulcerations of the esophagus, stomach, and small intestine (fatalities have been reported), and thus Indocin should not be given to patients with any sign of gastrointestinal distress (eg, peptic ulcer). Caution must be used in patients with epilepsy and parkinsonism because Indocin may aggravate these conditions and may also result in mental impairment making the performing of tasks requiring alertness (eg, driving a car) hazardous. The safe use of Indocin in pregnancy has not been established and the drug is not recommended for the nursing mother.

The most common side effects are headache, dizziness, nausea, and dyspepsia. Other CNS and gastrointestinal reactions occur, but less frequently. A large number of other untoward effects occur, but are of low frequency (see the package insert for details.) Among 205 patients on indomethacin studied in the Boston Collaborative Drug Surveillance Program, 21 patients experienced adverse effects as follows: CNS effects (9), gastrointestinal disturbances (9), dermatologic effects (2), and hematologic effects (1).

Indomethacin interacts with oral antacids, oral anticoagulants, beta-adrenergic blockers, thiazides and furosemide, lithium, and sympathomimetic amines (see Medical Letter reference).

LITERATURE Calin, A, Britton, M: JAMA 242(7):1885, 1979; Deodhar, SD, Sethi, R: Curr Med Res Opinion 6(4):263, 1979; Fox, IH, Kelley, WN: JAMA 242(4):361, 1979 (gout); Medical Letter 23(5):17, 1981.

INSULIN NPH
Isophane Insulin Suspension

1981: 78
1980:122
1979:136

Isophane Insulin Suspension is an intermediate-acting insulin preparation and, like other insulins, stimulates the cellular uptake of glucose, amino acids, and nucleotides. It also increases lipogenesis. Insulins are believed to act on a specific cellular receptor. Insulin NPH is given subcutaneously and has a peak action occurring 8–12 hours after injection. The duration of action is 18–24 hours. It is the recommended insulin in previously untreated diabetics. Highly purified insulins are now available that may be beneficial for patients with insulin allergy or resistance and also for those with lipoatrophy at the injection site. (See Medical Letter reference.)

INDICATIONS	Diabetes of all kinds, except for initial treatment of diabetic ketoacidosis or in emergencies.
PREPARATIONS	40, 80, and 100 units/ml in 10 ml containers for subcutaneous administration.
DOSAGE	The dosage must be individualized. Initially 10–20 units ½ or 1 hour before breakfast (30–40 units in obese adults). Not for intravenous use.
CONTRAINDICATIONS AND PRECAUTIONS	Known hypersensitivity to this drug or other insulins is a contraindication.
ADVERSE REACTIONS	Hypoglycemia is the most common side effect. Among 1194 patients receiving insulin in the Boston Collaborative Drug Surveillance Program, 109 patients had adverse reactions as follows: hypoglycemia (97), coma (5), hypokalemia (5), convulsions (1), and injection site complications (1).
LITERATURE	Larner, J: In The Pharmacological Basis of Therapeutics, 6th ed (Gilman, AG, Goodman, LS, Gilman, A, eds). New York, Macmillan, 1980, Chapter 64; Medical Letter 23:53, 1981 (on purified insulin preparations).

IONAMIN® (Pennwalt)
Phentermine resin

1981:159
1980:137
1979:123

Ionamin, an antiobesity compound, is a sympathomimetic amine with pharmacologic activity similar to that of the amphetamines. Besides suppressing appetite its actions include central nervous system stimulation and some elevation of blood pressure.

INDICATIONS	Ionamin is indicated in the management of exogenous obesity as a short-term adjunct in a treatment program based on weight reduction due to caloric restriction.
PREPARATIONS	Capsules: 15 and 30 mg.
DOSAGE	1 capsule daily, either before breakfast or 10 to 14 hours before bedtime. The 15 mg capsule is usually sufficient, but the 30 mg preparation can be used in the less responsive patient. This drug is not for use in children under 12 years of age.
CONTRAINDICATIONS AND PRECAUTIONS	Ionamin should not be used in patients with advanced arteriosclerosis, symptomatic cardiovascular disease, moderate to severe hypertension, hyperthyroidism, hypersensitivity or idiosyncrasy to the sympathomimetic amines, or glaucoma. The product should also be avoided in patients who are agitated, have a history of drug abuse, or are within 14 days of taking an MAO inhibitor. This drug may impair the performance of mental tasks requiring alertness and coordination (eg, driving a car), and because of the similarity in structure to amphetamine may result in intense psychic dependence and severe social dysfunction. Abrupt cessation of the drug results in fatigue and mental depression. Insulin requirements for patients with diabetes mellitus may be altered and Ionamin may decrease the hypotensive effect of guanethidine. The safe use of this compound in pregnancy has not been established; should not be used in children under 12 years of age.
ADVERSE REACTIONS	Cardiovascular effects include palpitation, tachycardia, and elevation of blood pressure. CNS overstimulation, gastrointesti-

149

nal disturbances, allergic reactions, and impotence can occur.

LITERATURE

Craddock, D: Drugs 11:378, 1976 (on anoretic drugs); Gershberg, H, et al: Curr Ther Res 22(6):814, 1977; Truant, Ap, et al: Curr Ther Res 14:726, 1972.

ISORDIL® (Ives)
Isosorbide dinitrate

1981:26
1980:32
1979:33

The basic action of Isordil (similar to that of all nitrates) is relaxation of smooth muscle. It is used in the treatment of angina pectoris. The precise relationship between this vascular relaxation and the clinical usefulness in the treatment of angina pectoris is not clear. The object of the therapy is a decrease in the frequency and the severity of the attacks of angina pectoris and a decrease in the need to use nitroglycerin.

INDICATIONS

Probably effective when taken by sublingual or chewable routes for the treatment of acute anginal attacks and for prophylaxis in situations likely to provoke such attacks. It is "possibly" effective when taken by the oral route.

PREPARATIONS

Sublingual tablets: 2.5 and 5 mg. Chewable tablets: 10 mg. Tablets: 5, 10, and 20 mg. Tembids tablets 40 mg; Tembids capsules 40 mg.

DOSAGE

Sublingual tablets: usually one or two 5 mg tablets every 2 to 3 hours. Chewable tablets: initially, 5 mg (½ tablet). For prophylaxis the lowest effective dose is taken every 2 or 3 hours. Oral tablets: usual range is 5–30 mg four times daily. Tembids (tablets or capsules): one every 6–12 hours.

CONTRAINDICATIONS AND PRECAUTIONS
Should not be used in patients with known sensitivity to this drug. Tolerance and cross-tolerance to other nitrates and nitrites may occur.

ADVERSE REACTIONS
Headache is the most common side effect. Cutaneous vasodilation with flushing occurs. Dizziness, weakness, gastrointestinal disturbances, and orthostatic hypotension occur. Among 361 patients on isosorbide dinitrate in the Boston Collaborative Drug Surveillance Program, 34 patients had adverse reactions as follows: headache (27), vertigo (3), gastrointestinal disturbances (3), and hypotension (1). This drug can act as an antagonist to norepinephrine, acetylcholine, histamine, and other agents.

LITERATURE
Battock, DJ, Chidsey, CA: Circulation 44:1147, 1971; Danahy, DT, et al: Circulation 55:381, 1977; Editorial: Am J Med 64:183, 1978; Poliner, LR, et al: Tex Med 73:53, 1977; Willis, WH, et al: Chest 69:15, 1976.

KEFLEX® (Dista)
Cephalexin

1981:15
1980:16
1979:15

Keflex is a semisynthetic cephalosporin antibiotic intended for oral administration. Cephalosporins are active against most gram-positive cocci and many strains of gram-negative bacilli.

INDICATIONS
Keflex is indicated as an alternate to penicillin for respiratory tract infections

151

caused by *S. pneumoniae* and group A beta-hemolytic streptococci. It is used for otitis media, for skin and soft tissue infections due to staphylococci or streptococci, and for genitourinary tract infections due to *E. coli*, *P. mirabilis*, and *Klebsiella* sp. It is also used for bone infections caused by staphylococci and/or *P. mirabilis*.

PREPARATIONS

Oral suspension: Packages of 1.5, 2.5, 5 and 10 g. After mixing as directed, concentrations are either 125 or 250 mg cephalexin per teaspoon (5 ml). Also available for pediatric drops which, after mixture, contain 100 mg cephalexin per ml. Capsules: 250 and 500 mg. Tablets: 1 g.

DOSAGE

Adults: usually 250 mg every 6 hours, but the range is to 4 g daily. Children: based on weight, usually 25–50 mg/kg body weight, divided into four doses. Higher daily doses, 75–100 mg/kg, are required in the therapy of otitis media. In the treatment of beta-hemolytic streptococcal infections, therapy should be continued for at least 10 days.

CONTRAINDICATIONS AND PRECAUTIONS

Keflex should not be used in patients who have shown hypersensitivity to cephalosporin antibiotics, and with caution in patients sensitive to penicillin. Caution should be exercised in patients with renal impairment. There is some evidence of cross-allergenicity of penicillins and cephalosporins. Safety in pregnancy has not been established.

ADVERSE REACTIONS

Diarrhea is the most common side effect. Nausea, vomiting, dyspepsia, and abdominal pain have also occurred. Hypersensitivity reactions occur. Anaphylaxis has also been reported. Genital and anal pruritis, eosinophilia, neutropenia, and cross-sensitivity to penicillins have been observed. Among 175 patients receiving cephalexin in the Boston Collaborative Drug Surveillance Program 17 patients had adverse reactions as follows: gastrointestinal disturbances (8), sensitivity reactions (5), and "other" (4).

LITERATURE

Bill, NJ, Washington, JA, II: Antimicrob Agents Chemother 11:470, 1977; Conference (various authors): Cephalosporins. Postgraduate Med J 46(Suppl):3, 1970; Medical Letter 24:21, 1982 (choice of antimicrobials).

KENALOG® DERMATOLOGIC (Squibb)
Triamcinolone acetonide

1981:130
1980:125
1979:125

Kenalog action stems from the anti-inflammatory action of the synthetic corticosteroid, triamcinolone acetonide. These creams, lotions, ointments, and sprays are primarily effective because of their anti-inflammatory, antipruritic, and vasoconstrictive actions.

INDICATIONS

For the relief of inflammatory manifestations of corticosteroid responsive dermatoses.

PREPARATIONS

Cream and ointment: 0.025%, 0.1% and 0.5%. Lotion: 0.025% and 0.1%. Also available as a spray.

DOSAGE

The creams and ointments are applied to the affected area two or three times daily. Rub in gently. The spray can contains directions for use.

CONTRAINDICATIONS AND PRECAUTIONS

Steroids are not to be used in patients with hypersensitivity to this class; this

153

preparation should not be used for ophthalmic purposes. The safety of this preparation in pregnancy has not been established and thus Kenalog should not be used in the pregnant woman for prolonged periods of time.

ADVERSE REACTIONS

Reactions are local and mainly occur with occlusive dressings. The following have been reported: burning, itching, irritation, dryness, folliculitis, hypertrichosis, acneform eruptions, hypopigmentation, perioral dermatitis, allergic contact dermatitis, maceration of the skin, secondary infection, skin atrophy, striae, and miliaria.

LITERATURE

Maibach, HI, Stoughton, RB: Med Clin North Am 57:1253, 1973 (topical corticosteroids).

K-LYTE® (Mead Johnson)
Potassium as bicarbonate and citrate

1981:145
1980:150
1979:145

K-Lyte is a tablet containing potassium as the bicarbonate and the citrate. It is used as a potassium supplement.

INDICATIONS

K-Lyte oral potassium supplement is indicated for therapy or prophylaxis of potassium deficiency. It is useful especially with the thiazide diuretics, corticosteroids, or in cases where severe diarrhea cause excessive loss of potassium. It is also useful when the dietary potassium is low. With careful monitoring, K-Lyte may be used for potassium replacement in cases of digitalis intoxication resulting in arrhythmias.

PREPARATIONS	Effervescent tablets: supplying 25 mEq or 50 mEq (K-Lyte DS) of potassium as bicarbonate and citrate.
DOSAGE	Adults: One 50 mEq (K-Lyte DS) tablet dissolved in 6 or 8 ounces of water once or twice daily, or one 25 mEq tablet dissolved in 3 or 4 ounces of water two to four times daily. These should be taken with meals and sipped slowly over a 5–10 minute period.
CONTRAINDICATIONS AND PRECAUTIONS	K-Lyte should not be used in patients with impaired renal function, hyperkalemia, or Addison's disease. It should not be used in patients with oliguria or azotemia. Patients with cardiac irregularities should be closely monitored and the tablet must be fully dissolved in order to avoid gastrointestinal irritation.
ADVERSE REACTIONS	Nausea, vomiting, diarrhea, and abdominal discomfort may occur.
LITERATURE	For a discussion of potassium supplements see McMahon, FG: Management of Essential Hypertension, Mt. Kisco, New York, Futura Publishing, 1978, Chapter 4.

KWELL® (Reed & Carnick)
Gamma benzene hexachloride (Lindane) 1%

1981:133
1980:120
1979:121

Kwell cream or lotion, is an ectoparasitic for scabies, head lice, and crab lice.

INDICATIONS	Indicated in the treatment of patients with scabies, head lice, and crab lice.

155

PREPARATIONS	Cream, lotion, or shampoo.
DOSAGE	For head lice, application of a sufficient quantity of shampoo (to thoroughly wet hair) is made to the affected and adjacent hairy areas and left in place for 4 minutes. Add small quantities of water to form lather. Rinse, towel dry and fine tooth comb. For pubic lice the shampoo is used as described above. For crab lice, a thin coating of lotion is applied to cover the hair and skin of the pubic area, and, if infested, the thighs, trunk, and axillary regions and left in place for 8–12 hours and then washed thoroughly. For scabies a total body application from the neck down is made. Lotion or cream is used on dry skin in a thin layer and rubbed in thoroughly. The medication is left on for 8–12 hours and is then removed by a thorough washing.
CONTRAINDICATIONS AND PRECAUTIONS	Should be avoided in any patient with known hypersensitivity to this product, and must be used with caution in infants, children, and pregnant women. Lindane penetrates human skin. It is also contraindicated in premature neonates.
ADVERSE REACTIONS	Exzematous eruptions have been reported. There is potential for CNS toxicity, especially in the young. Seizures have been reported. The incidence of adverse reactions is less than 1 in 10,000 patients.
LITERATURE	Coates, KG: Community Medicine, September 3, 1971; Lassus, A, et al: Dermatology Digest, December, 1975; Rasmussen, JE: J Am Acad Dermatology 5:507, 1981 (review on efficacy and safety); Shacter, B: J Am Acad Dermatology 5:517, 1981 (scabies and pediculosis). Solomon, LM, et al: Arch Dermatol, March, 1977.

LANOXIN® (Burroughs Wellcome)
Digoxin

1981:7
1980:7
1979:8

Digitalis glycosides, such as Lanoxin, increase the calcium pool needed for contraction, probably by the inhibition of Na-K-ATPase. Both the force and the velocity of myocardial contraction are increased, and the duration of systole is shortened. The refractory period of the A-V junction is increased thereby slowing the transmission of impulses between atrium and ventricle.

INDICATIONS

Lanoxin is useful in congestive failure, especially "low output" failure, as it increases force of myocardial contraction and increases cardiac efficiency. It also increases the refractory period of the A-V node and, thus, is useful in atrial flutter and fibrillation since it slows the ventricular rate that would normally accompany these arrhythmias. (Not indicated in sinus tachycardia unless it is due to failure.)

PREPARATIONS

Tablets: 0.125, 0.25, and 0.50 mg. Elixir pediatric: 0.05 mg/ml for oral use. For injection: 2 ml ampuls containing 0.5 mg. Pediatric injections: 1 ml ampuls containing 0.1 mg.

DOSAGE

Initial dose for adults and children (10 years or older): 0.75–1.5 mg; average oral maintenance dose is 0.125–0.5 mg daily. In the elderly patient, 0.125–0.25 mg is used for daily maintenance. Patients with renal insufficiency require smaller than usual maintenance doses.

CONTRAINDICATIONS
AND PRECAUTIONS

The presence of toxic effects (see below) induced by any digitalis glycoside is a contraindication for Lanoxin use.

Arrhythmias or conduction disturbances, especially ventricular premature beats, are common. A-V block has also been seen. Gastrointestinal disturbances, such as anorexia, nausea, vomiting, and diarrhea, are common. Central nervous system disturbances such as blurred vision, yellow vision, headache, and apathy are also seen. Among 3828 patients on Lanoxin observed in the Boston Collaborative Drug Surveillance Program 476 had adverse reactions as follows: arrhythmias or conduction problems (327), gastrointestinal disturbances (119), CNS toxicity (4), gynecomastia (4), injection site (I.M.) complications (3), electrolyte disturbances (5), and "other" (14). Digitalis effects are enhanced by certain diuretics and antagonized by certain oral antacids and by sulfasalazine and neomycin. In patients with hypokolemia, toxicity may occur even with serum concentrations of digoxin in the "normal range." Quinidine causes a rise in serum digoxin concentrations with the implication that digitalis toxicity might result.

LITERATURE

Aronson, JK: Clin Pharmacokinet 5(2):137, 1980; Drug Therapy 8:1, 1974; Fisch, C, Surawicz, B: Digitalis. New York, Grune and Stratton, 1969; Johnston, GD, et al: Eur J Clin Pharmacol 16:229, 1979; Marcus, FI: Mod Concepts Cardiovasc Dis 45:77, 1976; Smith, TW, Haber, E: Digitalis. N Engl J Med 289:945, 1010, 1063, 1125, 1973.

LAROTID® (Roche)
Amoxicillin

1981:138
1980:129
1979:134

Amoxicillin, an analogue of ampicillin, is a semisynthetic antibiotic with essentially the same broad spectrum of bacteriocidal activity as ampicillin against many gram-positive and certain gram-negative microorganisms. Like ampicillin, this drug is susceptible to destruction by penicillinase. It is stable in the presence of gastric acid and may be given without regard to meals. It is rapidly absorbed after oral administration.

INDICATIONS

Amoxicillin is indicated in the treatment of infections due to strains of the following organisms: gram-negative, including *H. influenzae, E. coli, P. mirabilis,* and *N. gonorrhoeae;* gram-positive organisms such as streptococci, *D. pneumoniae,* and non-penicillinase-producing staphylococci. Amoxicillin seems less effective than ampicillin for treating shigellosis. Infections of skin, soft tissues, lower respiratory, and urinary tracts caused by susceptible strains of the above microorganisms respond well to amoxicillin.

PREPARATIONS

Capsules: 250 and 500 mg. Oral suspension: each 5 ml of the reconstituted suspension contains 125 or 250 mg. Pediatric drops: each 1 ml of the reconstituted suspension contains 50 mg.

DOSAGE

Usual oral dosage range in adults and *children weighing more than 20 kg* is 250–500 mg every 8 hours. For children less than 20 kg, 20–40 mg/kg daily is divided doses at 8 hour intervals. The higher doses are used in lower respiratory tract infections. For uncomplicated gonococcal infections in men and women oral amoxicillin 3 g

159

plus 1 g of probenecid is given in a single dose, and in children *2 yrs or older,* 50 mg/kg amoxicillin plus 25 mg/kg of probenecid as a single dose.

CONTRAINDICATIONS AND PRECAUTIONS

Known hypersensitivity to penicillins is a contraindication.

ADVERSE REACTIONS

Nausea, vomiting, and diarrhea (less severe than with ampicillin) can occur. Hypersensitivity reactions including rash, fever, serum sickness-like effects, anemia, eosinophilia, and other blood effects have been reported. Anaphylactic reactions occur much less frequently with oral penicillins than with parenterally administered penicillins.

LITERATURE

Brogden, RN, et al: Drugs 9:88, 1975 (review on amoxicillin); Eichenwald, HF, McCracken, GH, Jr: J Pediatr 93:337, 1978 (review of antimicrobials); Medical Letter 24:21, 1982 (choice of antimicrobials); Neu, HC: Drugs 9:81, 1975 (editorial on new broad-spectrum penicillin). For treatment of gonorrhea in young children, see recommendation by Center for Disease Control: Ann Intern Med 90:809, 1979.

LASIX® (Hoechst-Roussel)
Furosemide

1981:5
1980:5
1979:5

Lasix, an anthranilic acid derivative, is a potent diuretic. It inhibits the reabsorption of sodium and chloride at both the proximal and distal tubules and also at the loop of Henle.

INDICATIONS

Oral Lasix is indicated for the treatment of edema associated with congestive heart failure, cirrhosis of the liver, and renal disease including the nephrotic syndrome. Lasix is especially useful when an agent of high diuretic efficacy is desired. It is also useful as adjunctive therapy in acute pulmonary edema. The intravenous or intramuscular administration of Lasix is indicated when a rapid onset of diuresis is desired, for example, in acute pulmonary edema or when oral medication is not practical. Another important use for Lasix is in the treatment of hypertension where it may be used alone or in combination with other antihypertensive agents.

PREPARATIONS

Tablets: 20, 40, and 80 mg. Oral solution: 10 mg furosemide per ml. Injectable ampuls: 2 and 4 ml with each ml containing 10 mg of furosemide; Prefilled syringes: 2 ml, 4 ml and 10 ml, each of concentration 10 mg/ml.

DOSAGE

Edema: In adults the usual initial daily dose is 20–80 mg given as a single *oral* dose. If needed, a second dose may be given in 6 to 8 hours. If the original dose is not satisfactory, increments of 20–40 mg may be made in subsequent doses carefully titrated up to 600 mg/day in severe cases. When doses of 80 mg/day or more are given for prolonged periods careful clinical and laboratory monitoring is needed. In infants and children the usual initial *oral* dose is 2 mg/kg body weight, given as a single dose. If necessary this may be incremented no sooner than 6–8 hours by 1 or 2 mg/kg, not to exceed 6 mg/kg body weight. The maintenance dose should be adjusted to the minimum effective dose.

Hypertension: The usual initial daily dose in adults is 80 mg divided into two

161

equal doses with adjustment to suit the individual patient. Parenteral administration is reserved for patients in whom the oral route is impractical or for emergencies. For edema 20 or 40 mg may be given intramuscularly or by slow intravenous administration (1 to 2 minutes). Consult the package insert for further details on parenteral administration.

CONTRAINDICATIONS AND PRECAUTIONS

This compound is not to be used in women with childbearing potential unless in life-threatening situations. It should not be used in anuria or in patients with hypersensitivity to this compound. Hypokalemia may occur and digitalis toxicity may be precipitated. Lasix should be used with caution in patients with hepatic cirrhosis and ascites, and not at all in patients with hepatic coma and states of electrolyte depletion. This drug should be discontinued if azotemia or oliguria develop during severe progressive renal disease. Patients with known sulfonamide sensitivity can show allergic reactions. Potentiation of the antihypertensive effects of other antihypertensive drugs can occur, as well as potentiation of peripheral or adrenergic blockers. Systemic lupus erythematosus may be exacerbated. Lasix should not be used in the nursing mother. Electrolyte depletion may occur; hyponatremia, hypokalemia, and hypochloremic alkalosis can result. Patients receiving salicylate therapy in conjunction with Lasix may experience salicylate toxicity at lower doses and lithium should not be administered concomitantly. Arterial responsiveness to norepinephrine may decrease.

ADVERSE REACTIONS

The extreme potency of furosemide can lead to dehydration, hypotension, hypokalemia, hypochloremic alkalosis, and a variety of gastrointestinal, CNS, hematologic, dermatologic, and other adverse effects. Dosage is very important. Furosemide interacts with a number of drugs including cephaloridine, chloral hydrate, corticosteroids, curariform agents, digitalis drugs, indomethacin, lithium, phenytoin, and propranolol (see Medical Letter reference).

Among 2705 patients on furosemide and studied in the Boston Collaborative Drug Surveillance Program, 283 experienced adverse reactions as follows: dehydration (106), hypokalemia (94), hyponatremia (26), uric acid elevation (15), gastrointestinal disturbances (8), neurologic disturbances (8), rash (3), hyperglycemia (2), and "other" (21).

LITERATURE

Barisco, CR, et al: Curr Ther Res 12(6):333, 1970 (comparison of furosemide in treating hypertension); Kleit, SA, et al: Am Heart J 79:700, 1970 (status of diuretic therapy); Levy, B: J Clin Pharmacol 19:743, 1979 (diuretics in C.H.F.); Saito, M, et al: Cardiovasc Res 10:149, 1976 (combination of furosemide and chlorothiazide in hypertension); Valmin, K, Hansen, T: Eur J Clin Pharmacol 8:393, 1976 (furosemide in essential hypertension).

LIBRAX® (Roche)
Chlordiazepoxide HCl
Clidinium bromide

1981:64
1980:53
1979:51

Librax combines the antianxiety action of chlordiazepoxide (see LIBRIUM) and the anticholinergic or spasmolytic effects of clidinium bromide. Clidinium is a synthetic anticholinergic agent which has been shown to have a pronounced antispasmodic effect and an antisecretory effect on the gastrointestinal tract. The anticholinergic action of clidinium approximates that of atropine sulfate.

INDICATIONS	Possibly effective as adjunctive therapy in the treatment of peptic ulcer and in the treatment of the irritable bowel syndrome and acute enterocolitis.
PREPARATIONS	Tablets: 5 mg.
DOSAGE	The optimum dosage varies with the individual. Usually maintenance is achieved with 1 or 2 capsules three or four times a day before meals and at bedtime.
CONTRAINDICATIONS AND PRECAUTIONS	Librax should not be used in glaucoma and in patients with prostatic hypertrophy and benign bladder-neck obstruction and in those with known hypersensitivity to Librium. Librax should not be used with alcohol or other central nervous system depressants and because of the effects on mental alertness, tasks requiring concentration and coordination (such as driving a car) should be done cautiously. Physical and psychological dependence including withdrawal symptoms may occur, particularly with patients who are prone to increase the dosage of their own accord. An increased risk of congenital malformation is associated with the use of this drug during pregnancy. The concomitant use of Librax with other psychotropic agents is not recommended, and particular caution should be exercised when combination therapy with MAO inhibitors or phenothiazines is used.
ADVERSE REACTIONS	The side effects seen with Librax are those of its components. Clidinium may pro-

duce typical anticholinergic reactions, ie, dryness of the mouth, blurred vision, urinary hesitancy, and constipation. For side effects and other information on chlordiazepoxide, see Librium.

LITERATURE

AMA Drug Evaluations, 4th ed. AMA and Wiley, New York, 1980, pp 991–1000; Head, HB, Hammond, JB: Am J Dig Dis 13:540, 1968.

LIBRIUM® (Roche)
Chlordiazepoxide HCl

1981:44
1980:36
1979:28

Librium is from the class of benzodiazepine antianxiety drugs. It has sedative, appetite-stimulating, and weak analgesic action. The precise mechanism is not known. In common with barbiturates, chlordiazepoxide blocks EEG arousal from stimulation of the brainstem reticular formation.

INDICATIONS

Librium is indicated for the relief of anxiety and tension, withdrawal symptoms of acute alcoholism, preoperative apprehension and anxiety, and as an adjunct in the treatment of various disease states in which anxiety and tension are manifested.

PREPARATIONS

Capsules: 5, 10, and 25 mg.

DOSAGE

The dosage should be individualized for the particular patient and the condition. Adults: for treating mild to moderate anxiety and tension, 5 or 10 mg three or four times daily; for severe anxiety and tension, 20 or 25 mg three or four times daily; for treatment of geriatric patients, or in the debilitated patient, 5 mg two to four times daily. When Librium is used to treat

165

preoperative anxiety the dose (oral) is 5–10 mg three or four times daily on days preceding surgery. (See package insert for parenteral use.) Children, 6 years of age or older: 5 mg, two to four times daily (up to 10 mg, if necessary, two or three times daily).

For the relief of withdrawal symptoms of acute alcoholism, the parenteral form is usually used initially (see package insert). If the oral form is used, the usual initial dose is 50–100 mg to be followed, if necessary, by repeated doses, up to 300 mg per day.

CONTRAINDICATIONS AND PRECAUTIONS

Librium should not be used with alcohol or other central nervous system depressants, and because of the effects on mental alertness, tasks requiring concentration and coordination (such as driving a car) should be done cautiously. Physical and psychological dependence including withdrawal symptoms may occur, particularly with patients who are prone to increase the dosage of their own accord. An increased risk of congenital malformation is associated with the use of this drug during pregnancy. The concomitant use of Librium with other psychotropic agents is not recommended, and particular caution should be exercised when combination therapy with MAO inhibitors or phenothiazines is used.

ADVERSE REACTIONS

Drowsiness, ataxia, and confusion are the most common. Other adverse reactions have been reported. Among 2086 patients on chlordiazepoxide in the Boston Collaborative Drug Surveillance Program 221 patients experienced side effects as follows: drowsiness (150), disorientation (20), vertigo, ataxia, nystagmus, or dysarthria (12), fatigue or malaise (8), CNS excitation (6), depression (5), respiratory depression (5), sensitivity reaction (5), hypotension (4), coma (1), and "other" (5).

Although infrequent, interactions with other drugs can occur: with alcohol, anesthetic agents, antacids, oral anticoagulants, anticonvulsants, barbiturates, MAO inhibitors, and phenothiazines.

LITERATURE

Frazier, SH (ed): McLean Hosp J 3:1, 1978 (the anxious patient); Gottschalk, LA, et al: In The Benzodiazepines (Garattini, S, Mussini, E, Randall, O, eds). New York, Raven Press, 1973, pp 257–280; Medical Letter 23:41, 1981 (choice of benzodiazepines); Sepinwall, J, Cook, L: In Handbook of Psychopharmacol 13 (Iverson, LL, et al, eds) New York, Plenum, 1978, pp 345–393.

LIDEX® (Syntex)
Fluocinonide

1981:132
1980:143
1979:148

Lidex is a steroid compound available in cream, ointment or gel form for topical use. Lidex preparations are primarily effective because of their anti-inflammatory, antipruritic, and vasoconstrictive actions.

INDICATIONS

Lidex is used for the relief of inflammatory manifestations of corticosteroid responsive dermatoses.

PREPARATIONS

Cream, ointment, and gel of 0.05%.

DOSAGE

A small amount should be gently massaged into the affected area three or four times daily as needed.

Topical steroids are contraindicated in those patients with a history of hypersensitivity to any of the components of the preparation. Treatment should be discontinued if irritation develops. Safety in pregnancy has not been established. Use with caution in the presence of infection and when treating children and infants, especially when used with an occlusive dressing (since systemic absorption may occur). Topical steroids are not for ophthalmic use.

ADVERSE REACTIONS

Burning, itching, irritation, dryness, folliculitis, hypertrichosis, acneform eruptions, hypopigmentation, perioral dermatitis, allergic contact dermatitis, maceration of the skin, secondary infection, skin atrophy, striae, and miliaria have been reported.

LITERATURE

Brogden, RN, et al: Drugs 7:337, 1974; Maibach, HI, Stoughton, RB: Med Clin North Am 57:1253, 1973 (topical corticosteroids).

LIMBITROL® (Roche)
Chlordiazepoxide
Amitriptyline HCl

1981:143
1980:166
1979: —

Limbitrol combines the antianxiety drug, chlordiazepoxide, with the antidepressant, amitriptyline. This drug is recommended by the manufacturer for increasing the rate of response over that which can be achieved when either component is used alone.

INDICATIONS

Moderate to severe depression associated with moderate to severe anxiety.

PREPARATIONS

Tablets: chlordiazepoxide 10 mg plus amitriptyline 25 mg, and chlordiazepoxide 5 mg plus amitriptyline 12.5 mg.

DOSAGE

Adults: 3 or 4 tablets (10/25) daily in divided doses (up to 6 tablets daily if needed) for initial therapy, with adjustment to smallest amount needed. Patients who cannot tolerate the larger doses may use 5/12.5 tablets.

CONTRAINDICATIONS
AND PRECAUTIONS

This preparation is not to be used in patients who are hypersensitive to benzodiazepines or tricyclic antidepressants, or with monoamine oxidase inhibitors. This preparation should not be used during the acute recovery phase of myocardial infarction. Because of the atropine-like nature of amitriptyline, this preparation should not be used in patients with a history of urinary retention or angle-closure glaucoma. Severe constipation may occur in patients taking anticholinergics in combination with Limbitrol. Arrhythmias, myocardial infarction, and stroke have been reported in patients receiving this class of drugs. The safe use of this preparation in pregnancy and lactation has not been established, and chlordiazepoxide has been found to increase the risk of congenital malformations. Physical and psychological dependence has resulted from the use of this preparation and withdrawal symptoms can occur following cessation of either component of this preparation (but not thus far with the combined preparation). Caution should be exercised in patients with a history of seizures, and those with hyperthyroidism, as well as those with impaired renal and hepatic function. Patients with suicidal tendencies should not have easy access to large quan-

169

tities. Limbitrol may block the antihypertensive effects of guanethidine or similar compounds. Limbitrol may be additive with other central nervous system depressants and may impair tasks requiring mental alertness (such as driving a car). Safety has not been established in children below the age of 12 years. In elderly and debilitated patients the dose should be reduced.

ADVERSE REACTIONS

The untoward reactions to this drug are those associated with the use of either component alone. Most frequently, drowsiness, dry mouth, constipation, blurred vision, dizziness, and bloating. Less frequently occurring are impotence, CNS effects, and nasal congestion. Rarely reported are granulocytopenia, jaundice and hepatic dysfunction. (See also ELAVIL and LIBRIUM)

LITERATURE

AMA Drug Evaluations, 4th ed. New York, AMA and Wiley, 1980, p 207; Medical Letter 20:49, 1978.

LOMOTIL® (Searle)
Diphenoxylate HCl
Atropine sulfate

1981:51
1980:46
1979:40

Lomotil depresses intestinal motility. Diphenoxylate is chemically related to the narcotic meperidine. Atropine is anticholinergic.

INDICATIONS

Lomotil is effective as adjunctive therapy in the management of diarrhea.

PREPARATIONS

Tablet: 2.5 mg diphenoxylate hydrochloride and 0.025 mg atropine sulfate. Liquid: 2.5 mg diphenoxylate and 0.025 mg atropine per 5 ml.

DOSAGE

Adults: initially 2 tablets four times daily or 10 ml (2 teaspoons) of the liquid four times a day (that is, 20 mg/day). Control may often be maintained with 5 mg (2 tablets or 10 ml of liquid) daily. Children, 2 years or older: should initially receive the liquid, not the tablet, based on weight: 0.3 to 0.4 mg/kg daily administered in divided doses. Control is often maintained with ¼ of this daily dose. (Not for children less than 2 years of age.)

CONTRAINDICATIONS
AND PRECAUTIONS

This preparation should not be used in children of less than 2 years or in patients who are jaundiced. In addition, Lomotil is not to be used for the treatment of diarrhea associated with pseudomembranous enterocolitis (which may occur during or up to several weeks following treatment with antibiotics such as clindamycin). Lomotil is also not indicated when the patient is known to be hypersensitive to diphenoxylate or atropine.

ADVERSE REACTIONS

Atropine effects such as dryness, flushing, hyperthermia, tachycardia, and urinary retention may occur, especially in children. A number of other reactions have been reported. Among 629 patients receiving this combination 27 patients experienced side effects as recorded in the Boston Collaborative Drug Surveillance Program as follows: constipation (17), other gastrointestinal disturbances (4), voiding difficulty (2), hepatic coma (1), hallucinations (1), fever (1), and drowsiness (1). Interactions with clindamycin and lincomycin can produce increased diarrhea. (See Medical Letter citation).

171

LITERATURE   Anon: Br Med J 4:606, 1969 (drugs for diarrhea); Barowsky, H, Schwartz, SA: JAMA 180:1058, 1962; Medical Letter 23:17, 1981; Rosenstein, G, et al: Pediatrics 51:32, 1973.

LO/OVRAL® (Wyeth)
Norgestrel
Ethinyl estradiol

1981:63
1980:65
1979:65

Lo/Ovral is a combination oral contraceptive preparation. It acts mainly through the mechanism of gonadotropin suppression due to the estrogenic and progestational activity of the constituents. The predominant effect of estrogen is to inhibit secretion of FSH, while continued action of progesterone (related, but not equated to progestins) is to inhibit LH. Alterations in the genital tract, such as changes in the cervical mucus and the endometrium, may also contribute to the contraceptive effectiveness.

INDICATIONS   For the prevention of pregnancy in women who elect to use oral contraceptives as a method of contraception.

PREPARATIONS   Tablets: 0.3 mg norgestrel and 0.03 mg ethinyl estradiol.

DOSAGE   One tablet daily for 21 consecutive days per menstrual cycle. One tablet daily starting on day 5 of the menstrual cycle (the first day of menstruation is counted as day 1) and continues for 21 days. Subsequent cycles begin on the eighth day after taking the last tablet, again starting on the same day of the week on which she began her first course. All subsequent cycles will begin on that same day of the week, that is, one tablet each day for 3 weeks followed by a week of no pill taking.

CONTRAINDICATIONS AND PRECAUTIONS

Oral contraceptives should not be used in women with any of the following conditions: (1) thrombophlebitis or thromboembolic disorders. (2) A past history of deep vein thrombophlebitis or thromboembolic disorders. (3) Cerebral vascular or coronary artery disease. (4) Known or suspected carcinoma of the breast. (5) Known or suspected estrogen-dependent neoplasia. (6) Undiagnosed, abnormal genital bleeding. (7) Known or suspected pregnancy. (8) Benign or malignant liver tumor which developed during the use of oral contraceptives or other estrogen-containing products.

ADVERSE REACTIONS

A variety of major and minor side effects have been attributed to the use of oral contraceptives. Of major concern are cardiovascular side effects and the induction or promotion of tumors. Cigarette smoking increases the risk of serious cardiovascular side effects from oral contraceptives and the risk increases with age and with heavy smoking.

An increased risk of the following serious adverse reactions has been associated with the use of oral contraceptives: thrombophlebitis, cerebral thrombosis, gallbladder disease, pulmonary embolism, cerebral hemorrhage, liver tumors, coronary thrombosis, hypertension, congenital anomalies.

There is evidence of an association between the following conditions and the use of oral contraceptives, although additional confirmatory studies are needed: mesenteric thrombosis, neuro-ocular lesions, e.g., retinal thrombosis and optic neuritis.

173

The following adverse reactions have been reported in patients receiving oral contraceptives and are believed to be drug-related:

Nausea and/or vomiting, usually the most common adverse reactions, occur in approximately 10% or less of patients during the first cycle. Other reactions, as a general rule, are seen much less frequently or only occasionally. Gastrointestinal symptoms (such as abdominal cramps and bloating), breakthrough bleeding, spotting, change in menstrual flow, dysmenorrhea, amenorrhea during and after treatment, temporary infertility after discontinuance of treatment, edema, chloasma or melasma which may persist, breast changes: tenderness, enlargement, and secretion, change in weight (increase or decrease), change in cervical erosion and cervical secretion, possible diminution in lactation when given immediately postpartum, cholestatic jaundice, migraine, increase in size of uterine leiomyomata, rash (allergic), mental depression, reduced tolerance to carbohydrates, vaginal candidiasis, change in corneal curvature (steepening), intolerance to contact lenses.

The following adverse reactions have been reported in users of oral contraceptives, and the association has been neither confirmed nor refuted: premenstrual-like syndrome, cataracts, changes in libido, chorea, changes in appetite, cystitis-like syndrome, headache, nervousness, dizziness, hirsutism, loss of scalp hair, erythema multiforme, erythema nodosum, hemorrhagic eruption, vaginitis, porphyria, impaired renal function.

The extensive use of oral contraceptives among women throughout the world has prompted many studies aimed at determining toxicity and other effects of these agents. The data have, in some cases, proved to be convincing whereas in others the associations between the drugs and the reactions have been neither confirmed nor refuted. The literature citation below gives a balanced summary and contains further references.

LITERATURE   Murad, F, Haynes, RC, Jr: In The Pharmacological Basis of Therapeutics, 6th ed (Gilman, AG, Goodman, LS, Gilman, A, eds). New York, Macmillan, 1980, Chapter 61; Woutersz, TB: J Reproductive Med 16:338, 1976.

LO/OVRAL® 28 (Wyeth)

1981:140
1980:181
1979: —

This preparation contains 21 active LO/OVRAL tablets and 7 tablets containing inert ingredients so that a tablet is taken every day. The dosage is one LO/OVRAL (white) tablet for 21 consecutive days followed by one inert (pink) tablet for 7 consecutive days. During the first cycle of medication the patient should begin taking the LO/OVRAL (white) tablet on the first Sunday after onset of menstruation. If menstruation begins on a Sunday, the first white tablet is taken that day. (See LO/OVRAL)

LOPRESSOR® (Geigy)
Metoprolol tartrate

1981: 40
1980: 55
1979:115

Lopressor, a synthetic beta-adrenergic blocking agent, is believed to have greater selectivity for the $beta_1$ adrenoreceptor than for the

175

beta$_2$ adrenoreceptor. Thus, the action of Lopressor is preferential in cardiac muscle. This preferential effect is not absolute, however, and at higher doses, metoprolol inhibits beta$_2$ adrenoreceptors located in the bronchial and vascular musculature. As a beta blocker, Lopressor is similar to propranolol; however, the greater selectivity of action for the beta$_1$ receptor may be therapeutically advantageous in some patients. The mechanism of the antihypertensive action has not been clearly established for beta blockers. Evidence suggests that inhibition of release of norepinephrine from nerve terminals and suppression of renin release may contribute to the hypotensive actions.

INDICATIONS	Lopressor is indicated in the management of hypertension. It may be used alone or in combination with other antihypertensive agents, especially thiazide-type diuretics.
PREPARATIONS	Tablets: 50 and 100 mg.
DOSAGE	The usual initial adult dose is 50 mg twice daily, whether used alone or with a diuretic. The dosage may be increased at weekly intervals until an optimum effect is achieved. The usual maintenance dose is 100 mg twice a day and may range to 450 mg per day. The safe use of Lopressor in children has not been established.
CONTRAINDICATIONS AND PRECAUTIONS	Should not be used in patients in which blockade of beta-receptors would aggravate existing or potentially serious maladies, including sinus bradycardia, heart block greater than first degree, cardiogenic shock, overt cardiac failure and, in general, bronchospastic disease. Because of a somewhat selective beta$_1$ activity, restricted use in bronchospastic disease is sometimes possible with a concomitant beta$_2$ stimulating agent. Caution is required in patients with diabetes mellitus, impaired renal, hepatic, or thyroid func-

tion, and those receiving reserpine-like drugs or digitalis. Major surgery is a controversial contraindication of beta-blocking therapy. Nursing should not be undertaken by women receiving Lopressor and the drug should be used in pregnant women only when clearly needed.

ADVERSE REACTIONS

Lopressor is a new drug and, thus far, reports of adverse effects have been mild and transient. These include tiredness and dizziness (10%), depression (5%), diarrhea (5%), other gastrointestinal problems (less than 1%), shortness of breath and bradycardia (3%), and bronchospasm (less than 1%). Other effects reported include pruritis (less than 1%), cold extremities, arterial insufficiency, palpitations, and congestive heart failure. Headache, nightmares and insomnia have also been reported. Peyronie's disease has been reported in less than 1 of 100,000 patients. Drug interactions are the same as those of propranolol. (See INDERAL)

LITERATURE

A summary with references, is contained in the Medical Letter 20:97, 1978; additional commentary is in the Medical Letter 21:21, 1979, and a discussion of drugs for hypertension is given in Medical Letter 23:45, 1981.

LOTRIMIN® (Schering)
Clotrimazole

1981:118
1980:136
1979:143

Clotrimazole is a broad-spectrum antifungal agent that inhibits the growth of pathogenic dermatophytes, yeasts, and *Malassezia furfur*.

INDICATIONS	Lotrimin cream or solution is indicated for the following dermal infections: tinea pedis, tinea cruris, tinea corporis, candidiasis, and tinea versicolor.
PREPARATIONS	Cream: 1% in 15 and 30 g tubes. Solution: 1% in 10 and 30 ml plastic bottles.
DOSAGE	Massage into the affected and surrounding skin areas twice a day, in the morning and evening.
CONTRAINDICATIONS AND PRECAUTIONS	In either form (cream or solution) Lotrimin is contraindicated in patients with a history or indication of hypersensitivity to any of its components.
ADVERSE REACTIONS	Erythema, stinging, blistering, peeling, edema, pruritis, and urticaria have been reported. Incidence of side effects is low (3.6% in one study, with only 0.6% dropouts).
LITERATURE	Clayton, YM, Connor, BL: Br J Dermatol 89:297, 1973; David, LM, et al: Curr Ther Res 15:133, 1973.

MACRODANTIN® (Norwich-Eaton)
Nitrofurantoin macrocrystals

1981:92
1980:80
1979:78

Macrodantin is effective in the treatment of urinary tract infections when due to susceptible strains of *E. coli, enterococci, S. aureus* and certain susceptible strains of *Klebsiella, Enterobacter,* and *Proteus* species.

INDICATIONS	For specific urinary tract infections as indicated above. It is bacteriostatic in low concentrations and is considered bactericidal in higher concentrations.

PREPARATIONS	Capsules: 25, 50, and 100 mg.
DOSAGE	Adults: 50–100 mg four times a day. Children: dose is calculated on the basis of body weight: 5–7 mg/kg/24 hours, given in four divided doses. (Do not use in infants under 1 month.) This drug may be given with food or milk to minimize gastric upset. Therapy should continue for at least 1 week and for at least three days after sterility of urine is obtained.
CONTRAINDICATIONS AND PRECAUTIONS	Patients with anuria, oliguria, or significant impairment of renal function have increased risk of toxicity because of reduced excretion of this drug. Also contraindicated for pregnant women at term, infants (under 1 month), and those patients hypersensitive to the drug itself or other nitrofurantoin preparations such as Furadantin.
ADVERSE REACTIONS	Gastric reactions are the most common. Sensitivity reactions may also occur. Hematologic and neurologic side effects may occur rarely. Among 173 patients receiving nitrofurantoin macrocrystals studied in the Boston Collaborative Drug Surveillance Program 22 patients had adverse reactions as follows: gastrointestinal disturbances (16), sensitivity reactions (4), and "other" (2).
LITERATURE	Conklin, JD: Antibiotics Chemother. 25:233, 1978; Gleckman, R, et al: Am J Hosp Pharm 36(3):342, 1979; Holloway, WJ: Delaware Med J 44:99, 1972; Miura, K, Reckendorf, HK: In Progress in Medicinal Chemistry. New York, Plenum Press, 1967, Vol. 5, pp 320–381.

MECLOMEN® (Parke-Davis)
Meclofenamate sodium

1981:149
1980: —
1979: —

Meclomen is a nonsteroidal anti-inflammatory drug for oral administration. Its mode of action, like that of other nonsteroidal anti-inflammatory agents, is unknown.

INDICATIONS	For the relief of signs and symptoms of acute and chronic rheumatoid arthritis and osteoarthritis. Meclomen is not recommended for initial treatment because of gastrointestinal side effects, including diarrhea which is sometimes severe. The safety and effectiveness of Meclomen in patients with rheumatoid arthritis of class IV (incapacitated) have not been established.
PREPARATIONS	Tablets equivalent to 50 and 100 mg of meclofenamic acid.
DOSAGE	For rheumatoid arthritis and osteoarthritis, including acute exacerbations of chronic disease, the dosage is 200 to 400 mg per day, in 3 or 4 divided doses, not to exceed 400 mg per day. The smallest dose that yields clinical control should be employed.
CONTRAINDICATIONS AND PRECAUTIONS	Not for use in patients with previously demonstrated hypersensitivity, and not for patients in whom aspirin or other nonsteroidal anti-inflammatory drugs induce symptoms of bronchospasm, allergic rhinitis, or urticaria. Use with caution in patients with a history of upper gastrointestinal tract disease.
ADVERSE REACTIONS	The most frequently reported adverse reactions involve the gastrointestinal system

(10 to 33%). Rash and headache occurred (frequency 3 to 9%); less frequently reported were edema, urticaria, pruritis and dizziness. Other reactions, with incidence less than 1%, were: gastrointestinal, renal, hematologic and dermatologic. Drug interactions may occur with warfarin, aspirin, propoxyphene, and with antacids.

LITERATURE — Medical Letter 22:111, 1980 (review).

MEDROL® ORAL (Upjohn)
Methylprednisolone

1981:155
1980:162
1979:168

Methylprednisolone resembles the natural glucocorticoids, hydrocortisone, and cortisone, but, unlike these, has minimal salt retaining properties. It is a potent and efficacious anti-inflammatory agent for disorders of many organ systems. Like other glucocorticoids, it can cause profound and varied metabolic effects, and modification of the body's immune responses to many stimuli.

INDICATIONS — Primary or secondary adrenocortical insufficiency, congenital adrenal hyperplasia, nonsuppurative thyroiditis, and hypercalcemia associated with cancer. It is also useful in the treatment of rheumatoid arthritis and other rheumatic disorders, collagen diseases, many dermatologic diseases, and allergic states that are uncontrolled by conventional treatment. It is also useful in severe or acute as well as chronic allergic and inflammatory processes involving the eye and its adnexa. Adrenocortical steroid treatment is complicated and more specific indications for usage may be found in more specialized sources.

PREPARATIONS	Tablets: 2, 4, 8, 16, 24, and 32 mg.
DOSAGE	The dosage is variable, depending on the patient and the disease under treatment. The following is a guide. Consult the package insert for details. Anti-inflammatory effect: 4–48 mg daily initially, followed by adjustment. The lower doses will generally suffice in situations of less severity. When the dosage is lowered or discontinued it should be done in small decrements over appropriate time intervals.
CONTRAINDICATIONS AND PRECAUTIONS	Systemic fungal infections. Smallpox vaccinations and other immunization procedures should not be given to patients who are receiving corticosteroids. Caution is required for use in patients with ocular herpes simplex, existing emotional instability, nonspecific ulcerative colitis, and those given concurrent aspirin for hypoprothrombinemia. (Consult package insert.)
ADVERSE REACTIONS	There are many potential adverse effects when corticosteroids are used. These are, in many cases, extensions of their pharmacologic actions and can involve fluid and electrolytes, the musculoskeletal system, the gastrointestinal system, and the central nervous system. Endocrine functions may be affected and ophthalmic and dermatologic reactions can occur. Among 296 patients receiving methylprednisolone in the Boston Collaborative Drug Surveillance Program 19 had adverse reactions as follows: Cushing's syndrome (5), hyperglycemia (3), superinfection (3), gastrointestinal bleeding (2), psychiatric disturbances (2), and "other" (4).
	The metabolism of corticosteroids is increased by drugs that induce certain he-

patic metabolizing enzymes such as phenobarbital, phenytoin, and rifampin.

LITERATURE   Azarnoff, DL: Steroid Therapy. Saunders,
Philadelphia 1975; Haynes, RC, Murad,
F: In The Pharmacological Basis of Therapeutics, 6th ed (Gilman, AG, Goodman,
LS, Gilman, A, eds). New York, Macmillan, 1980, pp 1470–1496. Selker, RG, et
al: Neurosurgery 5(6):773, 1979 (on alter-
nate-day steroid administration).

MELLARIL® (Sandoz)
Thioridazine HCl

1981:53
1980:57
1979:53

Mellaril, one of the phenothiazines, is effective in certain psychotic
disorders. It reduces excitement, hypermotility, abnormal mental
initiative, affective tension, and agitation through its inhibitory effect
on psychomotor functions. Unlike other phenothiazines, thioridazine
has minimal antiemetic activity and minimal extrapyramidal effects.

INDICATIONS   For the management of manifestations of
psychotic disorders: for the short-term
treatment of moderate to marked depression with variable degrees of anxiety in
adult patients. It is also useful for the
treatment of multiple symptoms such as
agitation, anxiety, depressed mood, tension, sleep disturbances, and fears in geriatric patients. It is used for the treatment
of severe behavioral problems in children
marked by combativeness and/or explosive hyperexcitable behavior and for
short-term treatment of hyperactive children who show excessive motor activity
with conduct disorders such as impulsiv-

183

ity, difficulty in sustaining attention and mood lability.

Tablets: 10, 15, 25, 50, 100, 150, and 200 mg; available in packages of 100 and 2000. Concentrates: 30 mg/ml or 100 mg/ml (containing 3.0% and 4.2% by volume alcohol, USP, respectively); supplied in bottles and packages of several sizes. Mellaril-S is available as a flavored suspension of either 25 mg/5 ml or 100 mg/ 5 ml supplied in pint bottles.

DOSAGE

Dosage is individualized according to the degree of mental and emotional disturbance. The smallest effective dose should be used. Adults: For psychotic manifestations the dose is 50–100 mg three times a day with a gradual increment, if necessary, to a total maximum daily dose of 800 mg. After control is achieved the dosage is gradually reduced to that necessary for maintenance. For short-term treatment of moderate to marked depression with variable degrees of anxiety in adults the usual dose is initially 25 mg three times a day. The total daily dosage range is 20 to 200 mg. Children: For children aged 2–12 the range is 0.5–3.0 mg/kg/ day. For children with disorders of moderate severity 10 mg two or three times a day is the usual starting dosage. For hospitalized severe cases, or psychotic children, 25 mg two or three times a day is the usual starting dosage.

CONTRAINDICATIONS AND PRECAUTIONS

Severe CNS depression, comatose state, and extreme hypertensive or hypotensive heart disease are the major contraindications. Precaution is necessary when treating patients with a hypersensitivity to phenothiazines. A potentiating effect is possible with anesthetics, opiates, alcohol, and other CNS depressants, as well as atropine and phosphorous insecticides. Not intended for children under 2 years of age.

ADVERSE REACTIONS   Drowsiness, pseudoparkinsonism and other CNS side effects may occur, but are not frequent. Dryness of the mouth and other autonomic effects may occur. Dermatitis and other skin eruptions have been observed, but are rare. Effects on the endocrine system have been described and ECG changes and hypotension have been reported. Rare cases of parotid swelling have been reported. Phenothiazines interact with barbiturates, guanethidine, levodopa, lithium, phenytoin, and propranolol.

LITERATURE   Baldessarini, RJ: In The Pharmacological Basis of Therapeutics, 6th ed (Gilman, AG, Goodman, LS, Gilman, A, eds). New York, Macmillan, 1980, pp 395–414. Carlson, BE, Sadoff, RL: JAMA 217:1705, 1971 (schizophrenia); Fann, WE, et al: Psychosomatics 15:117, 1974 (neuroses, anxiety, and depression); Kurland, ML: Dis Nerv Syst 37:8, 424, 1976 (neurotic depression); Lofft, JG, Demars, JP: Dis Nerv Syst 35:409, 1974 (psychoneurosis).

MEPROBAMATE

1981:89
1980:82
1979:74

Meprobamate is the most widely used of the class of propanediol carbamates, a class of sedative-antianxiety agents. Meprobamate's actions are similar to those of the barbiturates in clinical usage. There is no firm evidence of muscle relaxation other than that associated with its sedating action.

185

INDICATIONS	For the relief of anxiety and tension as an adjunct in the treatment of various disease states in which anxiety and tension are manifested. It is also used for the promotion of sleep in anxious and tense patients.
PREPARATIONS	Tablets: 200 and 400 mg. Capsules: 400 mg.
DOSAGE	The usual dosage range for adults is 1.2–1.6 g daily divided into three or four doses. Children over 6 years of age receive a daily dose of 25 mg/kg body weight divided into two or three doses.
CONTRAINDICATIONS AND PRECAUTIONS	Acute intermittent porphyria is a contraindication to the use of meprobamate as is known hypersensitivity to the drug. The use of meprobamate during pregnancy and lactation should be avoided.
ADVERSE REACTIONS	In large doses drowsiness is common. Gastrointestinal reactions (nausea, vomiting, diarrhea) may occur. Cardiovascular effects such as palpitation, tachycardia, arrhythmias, transient ECG changes, syncope and hypotensive crisis have been reported. Mild allergic or idiosyncratic reactions may occur. More severe reactions have been rarely reported. Other reactions, less frequently seen, are thrombocytopenia, leukopenia, dermatitis, urticaria, anaphylactic reactions, hypotension, blurred vision, weakness of the extremities, and paradoxical reactions of euphoria and anger. In the Boston Collaborative Drug Surveillance Program 153 patients on meprobamate were studied. Four patients experienced drowsiness. No other untoward effects were reported in this study.

LITERATURE   AMA Drug Evaluations, 4th ed. New York, AMA and Wiley, 1980, p 158; Champlin, FB, et al: Clin Pharmacol Ther 9:11, 1968; Nyquist, R, et al: Arch Phys Med Rehabil 39:683, 1958.

MINIPRESS® (Pfizer)
Prazosin HCl

1981:69
1980:83
1979:95

Prazosin is an antihypertensive agent. The exact mechanism of the hypotensive action of prazosin is unknown but may be related to its blockade of postsynaptic alpha-adrenergic receptors. Prazosin causes a decrease in total peripheral resistance.

INDICATIONS   Minipress is indicated in the treatment of hypertension. As an antihypertensive drug it is mild to moderate in activity. Evidence suggests that it is more effective when used with a diuretic in more severe cases. Prazosin is under investigation for possible use in the treatment of congestive heart failure.

PREPARATIONS   Capsules: 1, 2, and 5 mg.

DOSAGE   The dosage should be individualized. The usual initial dose is 1 mg two or three times a day. For maintenance the dose may be *slowly* increased to a total daily dose of 20 mg given in divided doses. (The usual maintenance range is 6–15 mg.) If a second antihypertensive (eg, a diuretic) is added the dose of Minipress should be initially reduced to 1–2 mg three times a day and then adjusted according to patient response. There is no

187

clinical experience on the use of this drug in children.

CONTRAINDICATIONS
AND PRECAUTIONS

Minipress is not recommended for use in pregnant women, except where the potential benefit outweighs the risk to mother and fetus.

ADVERSE REACTIONS

The most common reactions are dizziness (10.3%), headache (7.8%), drowsiness (7.6%), lack of energy (6.9%), weakness (6.5%), palpitations (5.3%), and nausea (4.9%). Other reactions associated with this drug are orthostatic hypotension, edema, gastrointestinal disturbances, CNS effects, genitourinary effects, and dermatologic reactions. When first taken, the first dose of prazosin can cause sudden collapse and loss of consciousness in patients with hypertension. (Medical Letter, 1978; 1978a)

LITERATURE

Lund-Johansen, P. Postgrad Med 58-(Suppl):45, 1975 (essential hypertension); McMahon, FG: Management of Essential Hypertension. Mount Kisco, New York, Futura Publishing, 1978, pp 277–290; Medical Letter 20(3):16, 1978. Medical Letter 20(20):90, 1978a; Medical Letter 23:45, 1981; Rasmussen, K, Jensen, HA: Br Med J 4:346, 1975.

The following references concern the use of prazosin in heart failure: Goldman, SA, et al: Am J Med 68:36, 1980; Mehta, J, et al: Circulation 59–60(Suppl. II):310, 1979; Packer, M, et al: Am J Cardiol 44:310, 1979.

MINOCIN® (Lederle)
Minocycline HCl

1981:144
1980:148
1979:152

Minocycline, a semisynthetic derivative of tetracycline, has the same clinical antimicrobial spectrum as that of other tetracycline analogues. In contrast to other analogues, however, its serum levels are higher and persist longer than many other preparations.

INDICATIONS

Tetracyclines are indicated in infections caused by the following: Rickettsiae, *Mycoplasma pneumonia,* agents of psittacosis and ornithosis, agents of lymphogranuloma venereum and granuloma inguinale, and the spirochetal agent of relapsing fever (*Borrelia recurrentis*). The following gram-negative microorganisms are also sensitive: *Haemophilus ducreyi, Pasteurella* species, *Bartonella bacilliformis, Bacteroides* species, *Vibrio comma* and *Vibrio fetus* and *Brucella* species (in conjunction with streptomycin). *Tetracyclines* are alternates to penicillin in treating infections due to: *Neisseria gonorrhea, Treponema pallidum* and *Treponema pertenue, Listeria, Clostridium, Bacillus anthracis, Fusobacterium fusiforme* (Vincent's infection) and *Actinormyces* species. Certain other gram-positive and gram-negative microorganisms may be treated with tetracyclines when bacteriologic testing indicates appropriate susceptibility. *Tetracyclines* are usually not useful in streptococcal diseases; they have been successfully used in the management of acne. Other indications are in the treatment of trachoma and in inclusion conjunctivitis.

PREPARATIONS

Capsules: equivalent to 50 and 100 mg of base. Oral suspension equivalent to 50

189

mg base per 5 ml. Powder: equivalent to 100 mg of base (for intravenous use).

DOSAGE

The usual oral dose in adults and children over 12 years is 200 mg initially, followed by 100 mg every 12 hours. Children 8–12 years: 4 mg/kg body weight initially followed by 2 mg/kg every 12 hours. For treatment of syphilis the usual dose should be administered for 10–15 days. Gonorrhea patients sensitive to penicillin may be treated with Minocin, administered as 200 mg initially followed by 100 mg every 12 hours for a minimum of 4 days. The intravenous dosage in adults is 200 mg followed by 100 mg every 12 hours (not to exceed 400 mg daily). Children over 8 years: 4 mg/kg body weight initially, followed by 2 mg/kg every 12 hours. Therapy with tetracyclines should be continued for 24–48 hours after disappearance of signs and symptoms. Streptococcal infections require at least 10 days of treatment.

CONTRAINDICATIONS AND PRECAUTIONS

Known hypersensitivity to any tetracycline is a contraindication. Caution must be exercised in patients with renal or hepatic problems. The use of tetracyclines during the last half of pregnancy (tooth development phase) may lead to permanent discoloration of the teeth of the offspring. Infants and children under 8 years who use these drugs can experience tooth discoloration.

ADVERSE REACTIONS

Gastrointestinal disturbances (nausea and vomiting) are the most common adverse effects; tooth discoloration (as described above) can occur. Less frequent adverse reactions include malabsorption, enterocolitis, photosensitivity and various sensitivity reactions. Superinfection, rise in

190

BUN and renal damage may occur. Other reactions occur, but are rare. Among 1172 patients on tetracyclines studied in the Boston Collaborative Drug Surveillance Program 73 patients had adverse reactions as follows: gastrointestinal disturbances (41), superinfection (9), rise in BUN (8), sensitivity reactions (8), injection site complications (5), and "other" (2). These drugs interact with oral antacids, bismuth subsalicylate, oral contraceptives, oral iron, methoxyflurane, and zinc sulfate. This drug seems to cause more transient reversible vestibular reactions than other tetracyclines. Because tetracyclines may depress plasma renin activity, patients on anticoagulant therapy may require lower doses of the anticoagulant.

LITERATURE

Am Acad Dermatol (Ad Hoc Committee on Antibiotics) Arch Dermatol 111:1630, 1975; Finland, M: Clin Pharmacol Ther 15:3, 1974 (commentary on tetracyclines); Johnson, AH: Semin Drug Treat 2:331, 1972 (adverse effects); Medical Letter, 24:21, 1982 (choice of antimicrobials); Siegel, D: NY State J Med 78:950 and 1115, 1978 (reviews on tetracyclines).

MONISTAT® 7 (Ortho Pharm.)
Miconazole nitrate

1981:65
1980:60
1979:68

Monistat 7 is a vaginal preparation. The compound has a broad antifungal spectrum. The pharmacologic mode of action is permeation of the chitin of the fungal cell walls.

191

INDICATIONS

Monistat vaginal cream is indicated for the local treatment of vulvovaginal candidiasis (moniliasis).

PREPARATIONS

A vaginal cream supplied in 1.66 oz. (47 g) tubes with a measured-dose applicator. Also available as vaginal suppositories each containing 100 mg miconazole nitrate.

DOSAGE

One applicatorful of cream is administered intravaginally once daily at bedtime for 7 days, or one suppository inserted intravaginally once daily at bedtime for seven days.

CONTRAINDICATIONS AND PRECAUTIONS

History or indication of hypersensitivity to this drug. Pregnancy, except when essential to the welfare of the patient.

ADVERSE REACTIONS

During clinical studies with Monistat cream for a 14 day regimen, 39 of 528 patients reported complaints that were possibly drug related: vulvovaginal burning was the most common and occurred in 6.6%; other complaints, such as pelvic cramps, hives, rash, and headache occurred rarely (less than 0.2%). During clinical studies with the suppositories the incidence of vulvovaginal burning, itching or irritation was 0.5%, while complaints of skin rash occurred at only 0.2% incidence. Miconazole can increase the effect of oral anticoagulants; its anticandidal effect is decreased by amphotericin B.

LITERATURE

Pasquale, SA, et al: Contraception 15:355, 1977; Pasquale, SA, et al: Obstet Gynecol 53:250, 1979; Sargent, EC, Pasquale, SA: J Reprod Med 19:67, 1977.

MOTRIN® (Upjohn)
Ibuprofen

1981: 6
1980: 9
1979:19

Ibuprofen, a proprionic acid derivative, is a nonsteroidal, anti-inflammatory agent that possesses analgesic and antipyretic activities. Its
mode of action, like that of other nonsteroidal anti-inflammatory
agents, is not known. Ibuprofen inhibits prostaglandin synthesis
which may explain its particular effectiveness in treating the pain
of dysmenorrhea and other mild to moderate pain.

INDICATIONS

Motrin is indicated for the relief of the
signs and symptoms of rheumatoid arthritis and osteoarthritis. It is used in the
treatment of acute flairs and in the long-
term management of these diseases. It is
also indicated for mild to moderate pain.

PREPARATIONS

Tablets: 300, 400, and 600 mg.

DOSAGE

Arthritic conditions: the range is 300–600
mg three or four times a day, not to exceed 2400 mg total in a day. In general,
rheumatoid arthritis requires higher
doses than osteoarthritis. If gastrointestinal symptoms occur the drug should be
taken with meals or milk. For treating mild
to moderate pain the dosage is 400 mg
every 4 to 6 hours as needed.

CONTRAINDICATIONS
AND PRECAUTIONS

Patients with hypersensitivity to this drug
or other nonsteroidal anti-inflammatory
agents, (eg, aspirin). Patients with nasal
polyps, angioedema and bronchospastic
reactivity. Close supervision is required
in patients with upper gastrointestinal
tract disease, severe renal impairment,
cardiac decompensation, hypertension or
coagulation defects. Not recommended
for pregnant or nursing patients.

The most frequent adverse reaction is gastrointestinal (4–16%), most often nausea, epigastric pain, and heartburn. Dizziness and rash are common (3% to 9% each). Other CNS, dermatologic, and metabolic reactions occur with an incidence greater than 1% as do tinnitus and fluid retention. Other reactions can occur, but their incidence is less than 1%: elevation in blood pressure, congestive heart failure in patients with marginal cardiac function, hematologic reactions, depression, insomnia, gastric or duodenal ulcer with bleeding, and certain hearing and ocular disturbances. (Interactions may occur with coumarin-type anticoagulants and with aspirin.)

LITERATURE

Chan, WY et al: Am J Med 70:535, 1981 (dysmenorrhea); Daymond, TJ, et al: Rheumatol Rehabil 18(4):257, 1979; Garg, SL, Johnson, MS: Clin Pharmacol Therap 31:229, 1982 (comparison with aspirin); Keet, JG: J Int Med Res 7(4):272, 1979; Medical Letter 21:81, 1979 (dysmenorrhea); Medical Letter 23:75, 1981 (prostaglandin-inhibitor analgesics); Oyemade, GA, Onadeko, BO: J Int Med Res 7(6):556, 1979; Saxena, RP, Saxena U: Curr Med Res Opin 5(6):484, 1978; Schweitz, MC, et al: JAMA 239(1):34, 1978 (gouty arthritis).

MYCOLOG® (Squibb)
Triamcinolone acetonide
Gramicidin
Neomycin sulfate
Nystatin

1981:50
1980:43
1979:42

The actions of Mycolog cream and ointment are those of its components. Triamcinolone is primarily effective because of its anti-inflam-
matory, antipruritic, and vasoconstrictive actions. Nystatin is anticandidal. The two topical antibiotics, neomycin and gramicidin, provide
antibacterial activity.

INDICATIONS

Possibly effective in cutaneous candidiasis, superficial bacterial infections, infantile eczema, lichen simplex chronicus, and other conditions accompanied by candidal and/or bacterial infection. Mycolog cream may also be effective in pruritus ani and pruritus vulvae.

PREPARATIONS

Ointment or cream: both supplied in tubes of 15, 30, and 60 g, and jars of 120 g (4 oz.). Each gram contains 100,000 units of nystatin, 2.5 mg neomycin base, 0.25 mg gramicidin, and 1 mg triamcinolone acetonide.

DOSAGE

Cream: rub into affected areas two or three times daily. Ointment: apply a thin film to affected areas two or three times daily.

CONTRAINDICATIONS
AND PRECAUTIONS

Viral skin diseases (eg, vaccinia and varicella), fungal skin lesions (except candidiasis), and hypersensitivity to the drug or any of its several components. Usage during pregnancy should be limited. These are not for ophthalmic use, nor in

195

cases in which the circulation is markedly impaired.

ADVERSE REACTIONS   Hypersensitivity to the neomycin component occurs whereas hypersensitivity to nystatin and gramicidin is rare. Local skin reaction can occur. Ototoxicity and nephrotoxicity have been reported.

LITERATURE   Kaidbey, KH, Kligman, AM: Arch Dermatol 112:808, 1976. Marples, RR, et al: Arch Dermatol 108:237, 1973.

NALDECON® (Bristol)
Phenylpropanolamine HCl
Phenylephrine HCl
Phenyltoloxamine citrate
Chlorpheniramine maleate

1981:70
1980:72
1979:72

Naldecon is used for the relief of nasal congestion associated with pollen allergy and minor infections of the upper respiratory tract. Naldecon tablets are compounded in order to produce controlled release. The actions are those of its constituents. Phenylpropanolamine acts similarly to ephedrine. Phenylephrine is a vasoconstrictor. Phenyltoloxamine is an antihistaminic as is chlorpheniramine.

INDICATIONS   For relief of nasal congestion and eustachian tube congestion associated with the common cold, sinusitis and acute upper respiratory infections. Also for relief of the symptoms of perennial and seasonal allergic rhinitis and vasomotor rhinitis.

PREPARATIONS   Sustained action tablets, syrup, and pediatric formulations of the following compositions:

196

	Tablet (total)	Syrup (per 5 ml)	Ped. Syrup (per 5 ml)	Ped. Drops (per 1 ml)
Phenylpropanolamine HCl	40 mg	20 mg	5 mg	5 mg
Phenylephrine HCl	10 mg	5 mg	1.25 mg	1.25 mg
Phenyltoloxamine citrate	15 mg	7.5 mg	2 mg	2 mg
Chlorpheniramine maleate	5 mg	2.5 mg	0.5 mg	0.5 mg

DOSAGE

The usual dosage for the syrup, pediatric syrup and pediatric drops is every 3–4 hours in the amount shown in the table below. The sustained-release tablets are administered on arising, midafternoon and at bedtime in the amount (single dosage) shown in the table.

	Naldecon Pediatric Drops	Naldecon Pediatric Syrup (teaspoon)	Naldecon Syrup (teaspoon)	Naldecon Tablets
3–6 months	¼ ml			
6–12 months	½ ml	½		
1–6 years	1 ml	1		
6–12 years		2	½	½ tablet
over 12 years			1	1 tablet

CONTRAINDICATIONS AND PRECAUTIONS

Hypersensitivity to the compound itself or to any of its several ingredients. Also contraindicated in patients with severe hypertension, severe coronary artery disease, those on MAO inhibitor therapy, patients with narrow angle glaucoma, urinary retention, peptic ulcer and during asthmatic attack. Use cautiously in patients with hypertension, ischemic heart disease, diabetes mellitus, thyroid disease, increased intraocular pressure, peripheral vascular disease, or prostatic hypertrophy.

ADVERSE REACTIONS

Drowsiness. Hyperreactive patients may display tachycardia, palpitations, head-

197

ache, dizziness or nausea and other reactions associated with sympathomimetics.

LITERATURE

For a discussion of cold remedies, including Naldecon, see AMA Drug Evaluations. New York, AMA and Wiley, 1980, Chapter 30.

NALFON® (Dista)
Fenoprofen calcium

1981: 82
1980: 87
1979:101

Nalfon is a nonsteroidal, anti-inflammatory antiarthritic agent. In addition to its anti-inflammatory properties, animal studies have revealed analgesic and antipyretic activity; its mode of action is not known. In patients with rheumatoid arthritis, the anti-inflammatory action of Nalfon has been shown to reduce joint swelling, pain, and the duration of morning stiffness. Patients hypersensitive to aspirin may experience adverse reactions to Nalfon; however clinical studies have shown Nalfon produces mild gi adverse reactions and tinnitus less frequently than aspirin. It is not known whether Nalfon causes less peptic ulceration than does aspirin.

INDICATIONS

Nalfon is indicated for the relief of the signs and symptoms of rheumatoid arthritis and osteoarthritis. It is indicated in the treatment of acute flares and in the long-term management of these diseases.

PREPARATIONS

Pulvules: 200 mg; 300 mg. Tablets: 600 mg.

DOSAGE

Rheumatoid arthritis and osteoarthritis: 300–600 mg three or four times a day. Adjustment of the dosage depends on the patient's age, condition, and changes in disease activity but should not exceed 3200 mg daily. This drug should be taken 30 minutes before or at least 2 hours after meals. Analgesia: For mild to moderate pain, 200 mg every 4–6 hours.

CONTRAINDICATIONS AND PRECAUTIONS
Not for use in patients with known hypersensitivity to this drug, aspirin, or other nonsteroidal anti-inflammatory drugs. It should not be used in patients with significantly impaired renal function and with caution in patients with a history of upper gastrointestinal disease. The safety of this drug in children, in pregnant women and in nursing mothers is not known.

ADVERSE REACTIONS
Gastrointestinal side effects are frequent (14%). Other reported effects include headache and somnolence (15%), dizziness (3–9%) and other nervous system reactions occur. Palpitations occur in 3–9% and tachycardia less frequently. Nervousness and asthenia have occurred in 3–9%. Other reactions are less frequent and involve the nervous system, skin, and special senses.

LITERATURE
Brogden, RN, et al: Drugs 13:241, 1977; Medical Letter 23:75, 1981.

NAPROSYN® (Syntex)
Naproxen

1981:41
1980:52
1979:67

Naproxen, a proprionic acid derivative, has anti-inflammatory, analgesic, and antipyretic activity. In patients with arthritis this compound reduces joint swelling, pain, and the duration of morning stiffness.

INDICATIONS
Naprosyn is indicated for the treatment of mild to moderately severe, acute or chronic, musculoskeletal and soft-tissue inflammation.

199

PREPARATIONS	Tablets: 250 mg; 375 mg.
DOSAGE	The recommended initial adult dose is 250 mg or 375 mg orally, twice a day, followed by adjustment up or down to achieve the clinical response in the particular patient. The upper limit is 1000 mg daily.
CONTRAINDICATIONS AND PRECAUTIONS	Hypersensitivity to this, or other nonsteroidal anti-inflammatory drugs (including asthma, rhinitis, or urticaria). Should be used only with caution and close supervision in patients having upper gastrointestinal tract disease, impaired renal function, or compromised cardiac function. Not recommended for use in pregnant or lactating patients.
ADVERSE REACTIONS	Gastrointestinal reactions are the most common: heartburn, nausea, dyspepsia, abdominal pain, constipation, stomatitis, diarrhea, vomiting, melena, and gastrointestinal bleeding. Gastrointestinal disturbances are seen in 1 in 7 patients. Disturbances of the CNS occur in about 1 in 12 patients. These are mainly headache, drowsiness, and dizziness. Skin reactions occur in approximately 1 in 20 patients and adverse reactions to special senses occur with the same frequency. Cardiac reactions occur less frequently (1 in 50 patients) and hematologic reactions are even rarer. Probenecid may increase naproxen effects.
LITERATURE	Berry, H, et al: Br Med J 1(6109):274, 1978; Diamond, H, et al: J Clin Pharmacol 15:335, 1975; Katona, G, et al: Clin Trials J 8(4):3, 1971; Medical Letter 23:75, 1981.

NEOSPORIN® OPHTHALMIC
(Burroughs Wellcome)

Polymyxin B sulfate
Bacitracin zinc
Neomycin sulfate

1981:121
1980:113
1979:120

Neosporin ophthalamic ointment contains three antibiotics. Polymyxin B is an antibacterial agent whose action is restricted to gram-negative bacteria. Neomycin has antibacterial activity in vitro against a wide range of gram-negative and gram-positive organisms. Bacitracin is an antibiotic whose actions in vitro works against a variety of gram-positive and a few gram-negative organisms.

INDICATIONS	Neosporin Ophthalmic is indicated in the short-term treatment of superficial external occular infections caused by organisms susceptible to one or more of the antibiotics contained in the preparation.
PREPARATIONS	Polymyxin B sulfate 5000 units, bacitracin zinc 400 units, neomycin sulfate 5 mg.
DOSAGE	Ointment: an application every 3 or 4 hours, depending on the severity of the infection. Sterile solution: 1 or 2 drops in the affected eye two to four times daily. In acute infections therapy may be initiated with 1 or 2 drops every 15–30 minutes with a reduction in this frequency as the infection is controlled.
CONTRAINDICATIONS AND PRECAUTIONS	Hypersensitivity to this drug or any one of its several components. Allergic cross-reaction may occur with other antibiotics.
ADVERSE REACTIONS	Cutaneous sensitization to neomycin can occur (Grant, 1974).
LITERATURE	Aronson, SB, Bettman, JW: In Combination Drugs: Their Use and Regulation

(Lasagna, L, ed). New York, Stratton Intercontinental, 1975, pp 96–109; Grant, WM: Toxicology of the Eye, 2nd ed. Springfield, Illinois, Thomas, 1974, p 744; Medical Letter 18(17):69, 1976.

NITRO-BID® (Marion)
Nitroglycerin
(Sustained release capsules and ointment)

1981: 77
1980: 89
1979:117

Nitroglycerin is the prototype antianginal drug. It relaxes arterial and venous smooth muscle including the large coronary arteries. The mechanism of its antianginal effect is complicated and is only partly explained by its coronary vasodilating action. More likely its effectiveness in the typical angina patient is due to reduction in myocardial oxygen demand secondary to reduction of cardiac preload and afterload which results in reduced cardiac output and ventricular wall stress.

INDICATIONS

For the management, prophylaxis or treatment of anginal attacks. There is doubt as to the utility of orally administered preparations of nitroglycerin (Goldstein and Epstein, 1973), although a more recent study (Davidov and Mroczek, 1977) reported a significant reduction in the frequency of anginal attacks and an increase in exercise capacity with sustained-release nitroglycerin capsules. The ointment has been shown to be effective in angina (Wayne, 1977; Abrams, 1977) especially in patients with nocturnal angina or associated LV dysfunction (Abrams, 1977).

PREPARATIONS

Controlled release capsules: 2.5, 6.5, and 9 mg. Ointment: 2% nitroglycerin.

202

DOSAGE	Capsules: the smallest effective capsule strength is used (swallowed) two or three times a day at 8–12 hour intervals under most circumstances. Ointment: applied every 3–4 hours as needed. The usual dose is 1–2 inches, as squeezed from the tube, although some patients require as much as 4–5 inches. The ointment is spread in a thin uniform layer on the skin, without massaging or rubbing it in. The optimum dosage is determined by starting with ½ inch of ointment and increasing the dose in ½ inch increments.
CONTRAINDICATIONS AND PRECAUTIONS	Acute or recent myocardial infarction, severe anemia, closed-angle glaucoma, postural hypotension, increased intracranial pressure, or hypersensitivity to the drug or to nitrites.
ADVERSE REACTIONS	Transient headache and hypotension and its consequences are the most common side effects with nitrites. Among 181 patients on *oral* nitroglycerin sustained release preparations studied in the Boston Collaborative Drug Surveillance Program, 14 experienced headache. In 11 of these 14 patients the drug was discontinued because of the adverse effect. No other side effects were reported in this group.
LITERATURE	Abrams, J: Angiology 28:217, 1977; Davidov, ME, Mroczek, W: Angiology 28:181, 1977; Goldstein, RE, Epstein, SE: Circulation 48:917, 1973; Medical Letter 23:82, 1981 (ointment); Wayne, H: Angiology 28:203, 1977.

NITROGLYCERIN

1981:59
1980:90
1979:91

Nitroglycerin is the prototype antianginal drug. It relaxes arterial and venous smooth muscle including the large coronary arteries. The mechanism of its antianginal effect is complicated and is only partly explained by its coronary vasodilating action. More likely its effectiveness in the typical angina patient is due to reduction in myocardial oxygen demand secondary to reduction of cardiac pre-load and afterload which results in reduced cardiac output and ventricular wall stress.

INDICATIONS

For the management, prophylaxis, or treatment of anginal attacks.

PREPARATIONS

Tablets for sublingual use: 0.15, 0.3, 0.4, and 0.6 mg. Sustained release capsules for oral use: 2.5, 6.5, and 9 mg. Ointment: 2% nitroglycerin. Transdermal ("band-aid"-type) products are available. These release the drug over 24 hours and are used for prevention and treatment of angina pectoris, but not for treating acute attacks. (See Medical Letter reference for further information on these products).

DOSAGE

Tablets: 1 tablet (0.15–0.6 mg) dissolved under the tongue immediately upon indication of an acute anginal attack or prior to engaging in activities known to precipitate such attacks (up to 3 tablets in a 15-minute period). Sustained release capsules: 1 capsule two or three times a day at 8–12 hour intervals is usually used. (Note: the lowest strength tablet or capsule that is effective should be used.) Ointment: application of ½–5 inches from the tube is applied (not massaged or rubbed in) every 3 or 4 hours.

CONTRAINDICATIONS AND PRECAUTIONS	Myocardial infarction, severe anemia, increased intracranial pressure, and hypersensitivity to the drug. Caution needed in patients with postural hypotension with closed-angle glaucoma, or with hyperthyroidism.
ADVERSE REACTIONS	Headache and gastrointestinal disturbances are the most common side effects; hypotension and its consequences also may occur. Among 1000 patients on sublingual nitroglycerin studied in the Boston Collaborative Drug Surveillance Program, 44 patients experienced side effects as follows: headache (27), gastrointestinal disturbances (7), hypotension (5), vertigo (2), and "other" (3). One case of hypotension was life threatening.
LITERATURE	A comprehensive review of angina pectoris and its treatment is contained in Angiology 28, March 1977; also: Medical Letter 24:35, 1982 (transdermal delivery of nitroglycerin).

NITROSTAT® (Parke-Davis)
Nitroglycerin sublingual tablets

1981:139
1980:155
1979:177

Nitroglycerin is the prototype antianginal drug. It relaxes arterial and venous smooth muscle including the large coronary arteries. The mechanism of its antianginal effect is complicated and is only partly explained by its coronary vasodilating action. More likely its effectiveness in the typical angina patient is due to reduction in myocardial oxygen demand secondary to reduction of cardiac preload and afterload which results in reduced cardiac output and ventricular wall stress.

INDICATIONS	For the management, prophylaxis, or treatment of anginal attacks.

PREPARATIONS	Tablets: 0.15 mg (1/400 grain), 0.3 mg (1/200 grain), 0.4 mg (1/150 grain), and 0.6 mg (1/100 grain).
DOSAGE	1 tablet, dissolved under the tongue or in the buccal pouch, immediately upon indication of an acute anginal attack with repetition of the dose at 5 minute intervals until relief is obtained. Smallest effective dose should be used. A tablet may also be taken prior to engaging in activities known to precipitate an acute attack.
CONTRAINDICATIONS AND PRECAUTIONS	Myocardial infarction, severe anemia, increased intracranial pressure, and hypersensitivity to nitroglycerin. Caution needed in patients with postural hypotension.
ADVERSE REACTIONS	Transient headache may occur immediately after use. Manifestations of postural hypotension may develop. Among 1000 patients on sublingual nitroglycerin studied in the Boston Collaborative Drug Surveillance Program, 44 patients experienced adverse reactions as follows: headache (27), nausea and vomiting (7), hypotension (5), vertigo (2), and other reactions (3). One case of hypotension was life-threatening.
LITERATURE	A comprehensive review of angina pectoris, including treatment with nitroglycerin is presented in Angiology 28(3), 1977.

NORGESIC® FORTE (Riker)
Orphenadrine citrate
Aspirin
Caffeine

1981:181
1980:158
1979:155

Norgesic is a combination with analgesic, muscle relaxant, anti-inflammatory and antipyretic properties. Orphenadrine citrate is a centrally acting brain stem compound with analgesic and some anticholinergic properties. It selectively blocks facilitory functions of the reticular formation. The actions of the other compounds are well known.

INDICATIONS	Norgesic is indicated for the symptomatic relief of mild to moderate pain of acute musculoskeletal disorders.
PREPARATIONS	Tablets: orphenadrine citrate 50 mg, aspirin 770 mg, and caffeine 60 mg.
DOSAGE	The adult dosage is ½ to 1 tablet three to four times daily.
CONTRAINDICATIONS AND PRECAUTIONS	Situations in which a mild anticholinergic action is potentially harmful (glaucoma, pyloric or duodenal obstruction, achalasia, prostatic hypertrophy, obstructions of the bladder neck, and myasthenia gravis). Caution is required for use in pregnant patients, and patients who might have a hypersensitivity to the drug or any one of its several components. Not recommended for use in children under 12 years of age. With prolonged use, periodic monitoring of blood, urine and liver function values is recommended. Concomitant use of propoxyphene may cause confusion, anxiety and tremors.
ADVERSE REACTIONS	Side effects seen with this preparation are those seen with aspirin and caffeine or those usually associated with anticholinergics. These may include tachycardia, palpitation, urinary hesitancy or retention, dry mouth, blurred vision, dilation of the pupil, increased intraocular tension, weakness, nausea, vomiting, headache, dizziness, constipation, drowsiness, and rarely, dermatologic reactions.

207

LITERATURE   Birkeland, IW, et al: Clin Pharmacol Ther 9:639, 1968; Gold, RH: Clin Therapeutics 1:451, 1978: Gold, RH: Curr Ther Res 23:271, 1978; Gold, RH: Clin Trials J (London) 15:145, 1978; Mok, MS, et al: Curr Ther Res 22:361, 1977.

NORINYL® 1 + 50-21 (Syntex)
Norethindrone
Mestranol

1981:176
1980:171
1979:175

Norinyl is a combination oral contraceptive preparation. It acts mainly through the mechanism of gonadotropin suppression due to the estrogenic and progestational activity of the constituents. The predominant effect of estrogen is to inhibit secretion of FSH, while continued action of progesterone (related, but not equated to progestins) is to inhibit LH. Alterations in the genital tract, such as changes in the cervical mucus and the endometrium, may also contribute to the contraceptive effectiveness.

INDICATIONS   For the prevention of pregnancy in women who elect to use oral contraceptives as a method of contraception.

PREPARATIONS   Tablets: norethindrone 1 mg and mestranol 0.05 mg.

DOSAGE   1 tablet taken each evening at bedtime for 21 days as follows: The initial cycle begins on day 5 and goes through day 25 of the menstrual cycle, counting the first day of flow as day 1. No tablets are taken for 7 days, then, whether bleeding has stopped or not, a new course is started of 1 tablet a day for 21 days. This institutes a three week on, one week off dosage regimen.

Oral contraceptives should not be used in women with any of the following conditions: (1) Thrombophlebitis or thromboembolic disorders. (2) A past history of deep vein thrombophlebitis or thromboembolic disorders. (3) Cerebral vascular or coronary artery disease. (4) Known or suspected carcinoma of the breast. (5) Known or suspected estrogen-dependent neoplasia. (6) Undiagnosed, abnormal genital bleeding. (7) Known or suspected pregnancy. (8) Benign or malignant liver tumor which developed during the use of oral contraceptives or other estrogen-containing products.

ADVERSE REACTIONS

A variety of major and minor side effects have been attributed to the use of oral contraceptives. Of major concern are cardiovascular side effects and the induction or promotion of tumors. Cigarette smoking increases the risk of serious cardiovascular side effects from oral contraceptives and the risk increases with age and with heavy smoking.

An increased risk of the following serious adverse reactions has been associated with the use of oral contraceptives: thrombophlebitis, pulmonary embolism, coronary thrombosis, cerebral thrombosis, cerebral hemorrhage, hypertension, gallbladder disease, liver tumors, congenital anomalies.

There is evidence of an association between the following conditions and the use of oral contraceptives, although additional confirmatory studies are needed: mesenteric thrombosis, neuro-ocular lesions, e.g., retinal thrombosis and optic neuritis.

The following adverse reactions have been reported in patients receiving oral contraceptives and are believed to be drug-related:

Nausea and/or vomiting, usually the most common adverse reactions, occur in approximately 10% or less of patients during the first cycle. Other reactions, as a general rule, are seen much less frequently or only occasionally: gastrointestinal symptoms (such as abdominal cramps and bloating), breakthrough bleeding, spotting, change in menstrual flow, dysmenorrhea, amenorrhea during and after treatment, temporary infertility after discontinuance of treatment, edema, chloasma or melasma which may persist, breast changes: tenderness, enlargement, and secretion, change in weight (increase or decrease), change in cervical erosion and cervical secretion, possible diminution in lactation when given immediately postpartum, cholestatic jaundice, migraine, increase in size of uterine leiomyomata, rash (allergic), mental depression, reduced tolerance to carbohydrates, vaginal candidiasis, change in corneal curvature (steepening), intolerance to contact lenses.

The following adverse reactions have been reported in users of oral contraceptives, and the association has been neither confirmed nor refuted: premenstrual-like syndrome, cataracts, changes in libido, chorea, changes in appetite, cystitis-like syndrome, headache, nervousness, dizziness, hirsutism, loss of scalp hair, erythema multiforme, erythema nodosum, hemorrhagic eruption, vaginitis, porphyria, impaired renal function.

The extensive use of oral contraceptives among women throughout the world has prompted many studies aimed at determining toxicity and other effects of these agents. The data have, in some cases, proved to be convincing whereas in others the associations between the drugs and the reactions have been neither confirmed nor refuted. The literature citation below gives a balanced summary and contains further references.

LITERATURE   Murad, F, Haynes, RC, Jr: In The Pharmacological Basis of Therapeutics, 6th ed (Gilman, AG, Goodman, LS, Gilman, A, eds). New York, Macmillan, 1980, Chapter 61.

NORPACE (Searle)
Disopyramide phosphate

1981:162
1980:164
1979: —

Norpace is an antiarrhythmic drug available for oral administration. Its actions appear to be similar to "Type 1" antiarrhythmics (eg., quinidine and procainamide); that is, it depresses automaticity, retards conduction velocity, increases the effective refractive period of cardiac cells, and has anticholinergic actions. This drug may, in addition to suppressing arrhythmias, be of value when given prophylactically after myocardial infarction.

INDICATIONS   Norpace is indicated (after electrocardiographic evaluation) for suppression or prevention of recurrence of the following cardiac arrhythmias: unifocal premature (ectopic) ventricular contractions, premature (ectopic) ventricular contractions of multifocal origin, paired premature ventricular contractions, and episodes of ventricular tachycardia. (Persistant ventricular tachycardia is usually treated with DC conversion.)

211

PREPARATIONS	Capsules: 100 and 150 mg of disopyramide base, present as the phosphate.
DOSAGE	The dosage must be individualized. The usual adult dosage is 150 mg every 6 hours (100 mg in persons weighing less than 110 lb). For patients with cardiomyopathy, 100 mg every 6 hours; in cases of severe renal insufficiency, 100 mg every 10–30 hours. The interval will depend on creatinine clearance (consult package insert). Safe use in children has not been established.
CONTRAINDICATIONS AND PRECAUTIONS	Cardiogenic shock, second- or third-degree AV block (if no pacemaker is present), or known hypersensitivity to the drug. Caution is required in cases of poorly compensated heart failure, in patients with a history of heart failure, in patients with glaucoma, urinary retention, prostatic hypertrophy, myasthenia gravis, conduction abnormalities (eg., sick sinus syndrome, Wolff-Parkinson-White syndrome and bundle branch block), cardiomyopathy, renal impairment, hepatic impairment, and in pregnant or lactating patients.
ADVERSE REACTIONS	The most common reactions are anticholinergic, dry mouth (40%) and urinary hesitancy (10–20%) being the most common during clinical trials. The following were reported in 3–9% of patients: constipation, blurred vision, and dryness of the nose, eyes and throat, urinary frequency and urgency; nausea, dizziness, fatigue, muscle weakness, malaise and gastric pain. The following were reported in 1–3% of patients: hypotension, CHF, conduction disturbances, shortness of breath, and chest pain; anorexia, diarrhea, vomiting, dermatologic reactions, and nervous-

ness. Other reactions, less than 1%, were reported but a causal relation was not established.

Other antiarrhythmic drugs, occasionally used concurrently with Norpace, have produced widening of the QRS complex and/or prolongation of the Q-T interval.

LITERATURE

Heel, RC, et al: Drugs 15:331, 1978; Koch-Weser, J: N Engl J Med 300:957, 1979.

ORINASE® (Upjohn)
Tolbutamide

1981:97
1980:97
1979:83

Tolbutamide is an oral hypoglycemic agent of the sulfonylurea group. These agents stimulate the islet tissue to secrete insulin with consequent improvement in glucose tolerance. It is particularly noteworthy that tolbutamide will not lower blood sugar in the human subject who has no pancreatic beta cells. There may be some inhibition of the release of catecholamines.

INDICATIONS

The principal clinical indication for Orinase is diabetes mellitus of the stable type without acute complications such as acidosis or ketosis. This is the form of diabetes that has been variously described as the relatively mild adult maturity-onset or nonketotic type.

PREPARATIONS

Tablets: 250 and 500 mg.

DOSAGE

The average starting dose is 1 to 2 g daily, with adjustment based on patient response. The total daily dose may be taken either in the morning or in divided doses through the day. (See package insert when transferring patient from insulin to tolbutamide.)

213

CONTRAINDICATIONS AND PRECAUTIONS	Not effective alone in juvenile or growth-onset diabetes of the unstable type. Should not be used in diabetes complicated by acidosis, ketosis, or coma; and in the presence of fever, severe trauma, or infections. Also contraindicated in patients with severe renal insufficiency and in pregnant women.
ADVERSE REACTIONS	Hypoglycemia is the most common reaction. Other reactions, less often seen, are gastrointestinal disturbances, headache, allergic reactions, and blood dyscrasias. Liver dysfunction occurs but is extremely rare. Among 762 patients on tolbutamide studied in the Boston Collaborative Drug Surveillance Program 7 patients had adverse reactions as follows: hypoglycemia (5), thrombocytopenia (1), rash (1). Certain drugs may enhance the action of tolbutamide and thus increase the risk of hypoglycemia. These include insulin, sulfonamides, oxyphenbutazone, salicylates, probenecid, MAO inhibitors, phenylbutazone, dicumarol, and phenyramidol.
LITERATURE	Carlstrom, S, et al: Adv Exp Med Biol 119:411, 1979; Crowson, TW, Kriel, RL: Ann Intern Med 92(1):134, 1980 (on hypoglycemia); Kolata, GB: Science 203 (4384):986, 1979 (controversy over study of diabetes drugs); Rendell, M, et al: Ann Intern Med 90(2):195, 1979.

ORNADE® (Smith Kline & French)   1981:72
Chlorpheniramine maleate   1980:67
Phenylpropanolamine HCl   1979:60

Ornade, a controlled release spansule, contains a nasal decongestant, phenylpropanolamine, and an antihistamine, chlorpheniramine maleate that has drying and sedating actions.

INDICATIONS	For symptomatic relief of nasal congestion, runny nose, sneezing, itchy nose or throat, and itchy watery eyes as may occur with the common cold or in allergic rhinitis.
PREPARATIONS	Spansule capsules: chlorpheniramine maleate 12 mg, phenylpropanolamine HCl 75 mg. Liquid (for children): in each 5 ml (teaspoon), chlorpheniramine maleate 2 mg, phenylpropanolamine HCl 12.5 mg, alcohol 5%.
DOSAGE	For adults and children over 6 years of age: 1 capsule every 12 hours. Liquid: adults and children over 12 years of age, 2 teaspoons every 4 hours. Children 6–12: 1 teaspoon every 4 hours; 2–6 years of age: ½ teaspoon every 4–6 hours.
CONTRAINDICATIONS AND PRECAUTIONS	Hypersensitivity to any of the components is a contraindication. Concurrent use of MAO inhibitors should be avoided. This drug should also not be used in patients with severe hypertension, coronary artery disease, stenosing peptic ulcer, and pyloroduodenal or bladder-neck obstruction. Not for use in treating lower respiratory tract conditions including asthma. Safe use during pregnancy has not been established. Use cautiously in patients with cardiovascular disease, glaucoma, prostatic hypertrophy, or hyperthyroidism or diabetes.
ADVERSE REACTIONS	Drowsiness and dryness of nose, throat, or mouth, insomnia, and nervousness may occur. Other reported side effects include gastrointestinal disturbances, difficulty in urination, anginal pain, palpitation, headache, hypotension, and CNS disturbances. Among 237 patients on chlorpheniramine studied in the Boston Collaborative Drug

215

Surveillance Program 5 patients had adverse reactions. These were drowsiness (4) and urinary retention (1).

LITERATURE   Frank, DJ: Curr Ther Res 6(3):158, 1964; Norman, PS: Postgrad Med 54:94, 1973; Rumack, BH, et al: Clin Toxicol 7:573, 1975; Spry, CJF: Lancet 1(7958):545, 1976.

ORTHO-NOVUM® 1/35-21 (Ortho Pharm.)

Norethindrone
Ethinyl estradiol

1981:180
1980: —
1979: —

Ortho-Novum 1/35-21 tablets are a combination oral contraceptive. Each tablet contains 1 mg of the progestational compound, norethindrone, and 0.035 mg of the estrogenic compound, ethinyl estradiol. These are available in a dialpak dispenser containing 21 tablets. For further information see ORTHO-NOVUM 1/50-21 and OR-THO-NOVUM 1/80-21 which are also 21-day regimens indicated for the prevention of pregnancy in women who elect to use oral contraceptives as a method of contraception.

ORTHO-NOVUM® 1/50-21 (Ortho Pharm.)

Norethindrone
Mestranol

1981:52
1980:47
1979:49

Ortho-Novum is a combination oral contraceptive preparation. It acts mainly through the mechanism of gonadotropin suppression due to the estrogenic and progestational activity of the constituents. The predominant effect of estrogen is to inhibit secretion of FSH, while continued action of progesterone (related, but not equated to progestins) is to inhibit LH. Alterations in the genital tract, such as changes in the cervical mucus and the endometrium, may also contribute to the contraceptive effectiveness.

216

INDICATIONS	For the prevention of pregnancy in women who elect to use oral contraceptives as a method of contraception.
PREPARATIONS	Tablets: norethindrone 1 mg and mestranol 0.05 mg. 21 tablets in a "dialpak."
DOSAGE	One tablet daily starting on day 5 of her menstrual cycle (the first day of menstruation is counted as day 1) and continues for 21 days. Subsequent cycles begin on the eighth day after taking her last tablet, again starting on the same day of the week on which she began her first course. All subsequent cycles will begin on that same day of the week, that is, 1 tablet each day for 3 weeks followed by a week of no pill taking.
CONTRAINDICATIONS AND PRECAUTIONS	Oral contraceptives should not be used in women with any of the following conditions: (1) Thrombophlebitis or thromboembolic disorders. (2) A past history of deep vein thrombophlebitis or thromboembolic disorders. (3) Cerebral vascular or coronary artery disease. (4) Known or suspected carcinoma of the breast. (5) Known or suspected estrogen-dependent neoplasia. (6) Undiagnosed, abnormal genital bleeding. (7) Known or suspected pregnancy. (8) Benign or malignant liver tumor which developed during the use of oral contraceptives or other estrogen-containing products.
ADVERSE REACTIONS	A variety of major and minor side effects have been attributed to the use of oral contraceptives. Of major concern are cardiovascular side effects and the induction or promotion of tumors. Cigarette smoking increases the risk of serious cardiovascular side effects from oral contraceptives and the risk increases with age and with heavy smoking.

217

An increased risk of the following serious adverse reactions has been associated with the use of oral contraceptives: thrombophlebitis, pulmonary embolism, coronary thrombosis, cerebral thrombosis, cerebral hemorrhage, hypertension, gallbladder disease, liver tumors, congenital anomalies.

There is evidence of an association between the following conditions and the use of oral contraceptives, although additional confirmatory studies are needed: mesenteric thrombosis, neuro-ocular lesions, e.g., retinal thrombosis and optic neuritis.

The following adverse reactions have been reported in patients receiving oral contraceptives and are believed to be drug-related:

Nausea and/or vomiting, usually the most common adverse reactions, occur in approximately 10% or less of patients during the first cycle. Other reactions, as a general rule, are seen much less frequently or only occasionally: gastrointestinal symptoms (such as abdominal cramps and bloating), breakthrough bleeding, spotting, change in menstrual flow, dysmenorrhea, amenorrhea during and after treatment, temporary infertility after discontinuance of treatment, edema, chloasma or melasma which may persist, breast changes: tenderness, enlargement, and secretion, change in weight (increase or decrease), change in cervical erosion and cervical secretion, possible diminution in lactation when given immediately postpartum, cholestatic jaundice, migraine, increase in size of uterine leiomyomata, rash (allergic), mental depression, reduced tolerance to carbohydrates, vaginal candidiasis, change in corneal curvature (steepening), intolerance to contact lenses.

The following adverse reactions have been reported in users of oral contraceptives, and the association has been neither confirmed nor refuted: premenstrual-like syndrome, cataracts, changes in libido, chorea, changes in appetite, cystitis-like syndrome, headache, nervousness, dizziness, hirsutism, loss of scalp hair, erythema multiforme, erythema nodosum, hemorrhagic eruption, vaginitis, porphyria, impaired renal function.

The extensive use of oral contraceptives among women throughout the world has prompted many studies aimed at determining toxicity and other effects of these agents. The data have, in some cases, proved to be convincing whereas in others the associations between the drugs and the reactions have been neither confirmed nor refuted. The literature citation below gives a balanced summary and contains further references.

LITERATURE

Murad, F, Haynes, RC, Jr: In The Pharmacological Basis of Therapeutics, 6th ed (Gilman, AG, Goodman, LS, Gilman, A, eds). New York, Macmillan, 1980, Chapter 61.

ORTHO-NOVUM® 1/50-28 (Ortho Pharm.)
Norethindrone
Mestranol

1981:136
1980:154
1979:189

Ortho-Novum is a combination oral contraceptive preparation. It acts mainly through the mechanism of gonadotropin suppression due to the estrogenic and progestational activity of the constituents.

The predominant effect of estrogen is to inhibit secretion of FSH, while continued action of progesterone (related, but not equated to progestins) is to inhibit LH. Alterations in the genital tract, such as changes in the cervical mucus and the endometrium, may also contribute to the contraceptive effectiveness.

INDICATIONS	For the prevention of pregnancy in women who elect to use oral contraceptives as a method of contraception.
PREPARATIONS	Tablets: norethindrone 1 mg and mestranol 0.05 mg. 21 tablets (yellow) plus 7 (green) tablets containing inert ingredients in a "dialpack."
DOSAGE	The first yellow tablet is taken on the first Sunday after menstruation begins. If the period begins on Sunday the first tablet is taken that day. Tablets are taken without interruption as follows: 1 yellow tablet for 21 days then 1 green tablet for 7 days. After these 28 tablets have been taken, a yellow is then taken, etc.
CONTRAINDICATIONS AND PRECAUTIONS	Oral contraceptives should not be used in women with any of the following conditions: (1) Thrombophlebitis or thromboembolic disorders. (2) A past history of deep vein thrombophlebitis or thromboembolic disorders. (3) Cerebral vascular or coronary artery disease. (4) Known or suspected carcinoma of the breast. (5) Known or suspected estrogen-dependent neoplasia. (6) Undiagnosed, abnormal genital bleeding. (7) Known or suspected pregnancy. (8) Benign or malignant liver tumor which developed during the use of oral contraceptives or other estrogen-containing products.
ADVERSE REACTIONS	A variety of major and minor side effects have been attributed to the use of oral

contraceptives. Of major concern are cardiovascular side effects and the induction or promotion of tumors. Cigarette smoking increases the risk of serious cardiovascular side effects from oral contraceptives and the risk increases with age and with heavy smoking.

An increased risk of the following serious adverse reactions has been associated with the use of oral contraceptives: thrombophlebitis, pulmonary embolism, coronary thrombosis, cerebral thrombosis, cerebral hemorrhage, hypertension, gallbladder disease, liver tumors, congenital anomalies.

There is evidence of an association between the following conditions and the use of oral contraceptives, although additional confirmatory studies are needed: mesenteric thrombosis, neuro-ocular lesions, e.g., retinal thrombosis and optic neuritis.

The following adverse reactions have been reported in patients receiving oral contraceptives and are believed to be durg-related:

Nausea and/or vomiting, usually the most common adverse reactions, occur in approximately 10% or less of patients during the first cycle. Other reactions, as a general rule, are seen much less frequently or only occasionally: gastrointestinal symptoms (such as abdominal cramps and bloating), breakthrough bleeding, spotting, change in menstrual flow, dysmenorrhea, amenorrhea during and after treatment, temporary infertility after discontinuance of treatment, edema, chloasma or melasma which may persist, breast changes: tenderness, enlargement, and secretion, change in weight (increase or decrease), change in cervical erosion and cervical secretion, possible diminution in lactation when given immediately postpartum, cholestatic jaundice, migraine, increase in size of uterine leiomyomata, rash (allergic), mental depression, reduced tolerance to carbohydrates, vaginal candidiasis, change in corneal curvature (steepening), intolerance to contact lenses.

The following adverse reactions have been reported in users of oral contraceptives, and the association has been neither confirmed nor refuted: premenstrual-like syndrome, cataracts, changes in libido, chorea, changes in appetite, cystitis-like syndrome, headache, nervousness, dizziness, hirsutism, loss of scalp hair, erythema multiforme, erythema nodosum, hemorrhagic eruption, vaginitis, porphyria, impaired renal function.

The extensive use of oral contraceptives among women throughout the world has prompted many studies aimed at determining toxicity and other effects of these agents. The data have, in some cases, proved to be convincing whereas in others the associations between the drugs and the reactions have been neither confirmed nor refuted. The literature citation below gives a balanced summary and contains further references.

LITERATURE

Murad, F, Haynes, RC, Jr: In The Pharmacological Basis of Therapeutics, 6th ed (Gilman, AG, Goodman, LS, Gilman, A, eds). New York, Macmillan, 1980, Chapter 61.

ORTHO-NOVUM® 1/80-21 (Ortho Pharm.)
Norethindrone
Mestranol

1981:170
1980:135
1979:118

Ortho-Novum is a combination oral contraceptive preparation. It acts mainly through the mechanism of gonadotropin suppression due to the estrogenic and progestational activity of the constituents. The predominant effect of estrogen is to inhibit secretion of FSH, while continued action of progesterone (related, but not equated to progestins) is to inhibit LH. Alterations in the genital tract, such as changes in the cervical mucus and the endometrium, may also contribute to the contraceptive effectiveness.

INDICATIONS	For the prevention of pregnancy in women who elect to use oral contraceptives as a method of contraception.
PREPARATIONS	Tablets: norethindrone 1 mg and mestranol 0.08 mg. 21 tablets in a "dialpak."
DOSAGE	One tablet daily starting on day 5 of her menstrual cycle (the first day of menstruation is counted as day 1) and continues for 21 days. Subsequent cycles begin on the eighth day after taking her last tablet, again starting on the same day of the week on which she began her first course. All subsequent cycles will begin on that same day of the week, that is, 1 tablet each day for 3 weeks followed by a week of no pill taking.
CONTRAINDICATIONS AND PRECAUTIONS	Oral contraceptives should not be used in women with any of the following conditions: (1) Thrombophlebitis or thromboembolic disorders. (2) A past history of deep vein thrombophlebitis or thromboembolic disorders. (3) Cerebral vascular or coronary artery disease. (4) Known or suspected carcinoma of the breast. (5)

223

Known or suspected estrogen-dependent neoplasia. (6) Undiagnosed, abnormal genital bleeding. (7) Known or suspected pregnancy. (8) Benign or malignant liver tumor which developed during the use of oral contraceptives or other estrogen-containing products.

ADVERSE REACTIONS

A variety of major and minor side effects have been attributed to the use of oral contraceptives. Of major concern are cardiovascular side effects and the induction or promotion of tumors. Cigarette smoking increases the risk of serious cardiovascular side effects from oral contraceptives and the risk increases with age and with heavy smoking.

An increased risk of the following serious adverse reactions has been associated with the use of oral contraceptives: thrombophlebitis, pulmonary embolism, coronary thrombosis, cerebral thrombosis, cerebral hemorrhage, hypertension, gallbladder disease, liver tumors, congenital anomalies.

There is evidence of an association between the following conditions and the use of oral contraceptives, although additional confirmatory studies are needed: mesenteric thrombosis, neuro-ocular lesions, e.g., retinal thrombosis and optic neuritis.

The following adverse reactions have been reported in patients receiving oral contraceptives and are believed to be drug-related:

Nausea and/or vomiting, usually the most common adverse reactions, occur in approximately 10% or less of patients during the first cycle. Other reactions, as a general rule, are seen much less frequently or only occasionally: gastrointestinal symptoms (such as abdominal cramps and bloating), breakthrough bleeding, spotting, change in menstrual flow, dysmenorrhea, amenorrhea during and after treatment, temporary infertility after discontinuance of treatment, edema, chloasma or melasma which may persist, breast changes: tenderness, enlargement, and secretion, change in weight (increase or decrease), change in cervical erosion and cervical secretion, possible diminution in lactation when given immediately postpartum, cholestatic jaundice, migraine, increase in size of uterine leiomyomata, rash (allergic), mental depression, reduced tolerance to carbohydrates, vaginal candidiasis, change in corneal curvature (steepening), intolerance to contact lenses.

The following adverse reactions have been reported in users of oral contraceptives, and the association has been neither confirmed nor refuted: premenstrual-like syndrome, cataracts, changes in libido, chorea, changes in appetite, cystitis-like syndrome, headache, nervousness, dizziness, hirsutism, loss of scalp hair, erythema multiforme, erythema nodosum, hemorrhagic eruption, vaginitis, porphyria, impaired renal function.

The extensive use of oral contraceptives among women throughout the world has prompted many studies aimed at determining toxicity and other effects of these agents. The data have, in some cases, proved to be convincing whereas in others the associations between the drugs and the reactions have been neither confirmed nor refuted. The literature citation below gives a balanced summary and contains further references.

225

LITERATURE   Murad, F, Haynes, RC, Jr: In The Pharma-
              cological Basis of Therapeutics, 6th ed
              (Gilman, AG, Goodman, LS, Gilman, A,
              eds). New York, Macmillan, 1980, Chap-
              ter 61.

OVRAL® (Wyeth)   1981:58
Norgestrel   1980:51
Ethinyl estradiol   1979:45

Ovral is a combination oral contraceptive preparation. It acts mainly
through the mechanism of gonadotropin suppression due to the
estrogenic and progestational activity of the constituents. The predominant effect of estrogen is to inhibit secretion of FSH, while
continued action of progesterone (related, but not equated to progestins) is to inhibit LH. Alterations in the genital tract, such as
changes in the cervical mucus and the endometrium, may also contribute to the contraceptive effectiveness.

INDICATIONS   For the prevention of pregnancy in
                  women who elect to use oral contracep-
                  tives as a method of contraception.

PREPARATIONS   Tablets: norgestrol 0.5 mg and ethinyl es-
                  tradiol 0.05 mg (21 tablet container).

DOSAGE   1 tablet daily for 21 consecutive days as
                  follows: One tablet daily starting on day
                  5 of her menstrual cycle (the first day of
                  menstruation is counted as day 1) and
                  continues for 21 days. Subsequent cycles
                  begin on the eighth day after taking her
                  last tablet, again starting on the same day
                  of the week on which she began her first
                  course. All subsequent cycles will begin
                  on that same day of the week, that is 1

tablet each day for 3 weeks followed by a week of no pill taking.

Oral contraceptives should not be used in women with any of the following conditions: (1) Thrombophlebitis or thromboembolic disorders. (2) A past history of deep vein thrombophlebitis or thromboembolic disorders. (3) Cerebral vascular or coronary artery disease. (4) Known or suspected carcinoma of the breast. (5) Known or suspected estrogen-dependent neoplasia. (6) Undiagnosed, abnormal genital bleeding. (7) Known or suspected pregnancy. (8) Benign or malignant liver tumor which developed during the use of oral contraceptives or other estrogen-containing products.

ADVERSE REACTIONS

A variety of major and minor side effects have been attributed to the use of oral contraceptives. Of major concern are cardiovascular side effects and the induction or promotion of tumors. Cigarette smoking increases the risk of serious cardiovascular side effects from oral contraceptives and the risk increases with age and with heavy smoking.

An increased risk of the following serious adverse reactions has been associated with the use of oral contraceptives: thrombophlebitis, pulmonary embolism, coronary thrombosis, cerebral thrombosis, cerebral hemorrhage, hypertension, gallbladder disease, liver tumors, congenital anomalies.

There is evidence of an association between the following conditions and the use of oral contraceptives, although additional confirmatory studies are needed: mesenteric thrombosis, neuro-ocular lesions, e.g., retinal thrombosis and optic neuritis.

227

The following adverse reactions have been reported in patients receiving oral contraceptives and are believed to be drug-related:

Nausea and/or vomiting, usually the most common adverse reactions, occur in approximately 10% or less of patients during the first cycle. Other reactions, as a general rule, are seen much less frequently or only occasionally: gastrointestinal symptoms (such as abdominal cramps and bloating), breakthrough bleeding, spotting, change in menstrual flow, dysmenorrhea, amenorrhea during and after treatment, temporary infertility after discontinuance of treatment, edema, chloasma or melasma which may persist, breast changes: tenderness, enlargement, and secretion, change in weight (increase or decrease), change in cervical erosion and cervical secretion, possible diminution in lactation when given immediately postpartum, cholestatic jaundice, migraine, increase in size of uterine leiomyomata, rash (allergic), mental depression, reduced tolerance to carbohydrates, vaginal candidiasis, change in corneal curvature (steepening), intolerance to contact lenses.

The following adverse reactions have been reported in users of oral contraceptives, and the association has been neither confirmed nor refuted: premenstrual-like syndrome, cataracts, changes in libido, chorea, changes in appetite, cystitis-like syndrome, headache, nervousness, dizziness, hirsutism, loss of scalp hair, erythema multiforme, erythema nodosum, hemorrhagic eruption, vaginitis, porphyria, impaired renal function.

The extensive use of oral contraceptives among women throughout the world has prompted many studies aimed at determining toxicity and other effects of these agents. The data have, in some cases, proved to be convincing whereas in others the associations between the drugs and the reactions have been neither confirmed nor refuted. The literature citation below gives a balanced summary and contains further references.

LITERATURE

Murad, F, Haynes, RC, Jr: In The Pharmacological Basis of Therapeutics, 6th ed (Gilman, AG, Goodman, LS, Gilman, A, eds). New York, Macmillan, 1980, Chapter 61. See also Korba, VD, Heil, C: Fertility and Sterility 26:973, 1975.

OVRAL® 28 (Wyeth)
Norgestrel
Ethinyl estradiol

1981:197
1980:200
1979:193

This preparation contains 21 active OVRAL tablets and 7 tablets containing inert ingredients so that a tablet is taken every day. The dosage is one (white) OVRAL tablet daily for 21 consecutive days followed by one (pink) inert tablet daily for 7 consecutive days. During the first cycle the patient begins taking the white tablet on the first Sunday after the onset of menstruation. If menstruation begins on a Sunday, the first white tablet is taken that day. (See OVRAL)

CONTRAINDICATIONS
AND PRECAUTIONS

Oral contraceptives should not be used in women with any of the following conditions: (1) Thrombophlebitis or thromboembolic disorders. (2) A past history of deep vein thrombophlebitis or thromboembolic disorders. (3) Cerebral vascular or coronary artery disease. (4) Known or suspected carcinoma of the breast. (5) Known or suspected estrogen-dependent neoplasia. (6) Undiagnosed, abnormal genital bleeding. (7) Known or suspected pregnancy. (8) Benign or malignant liver tumor which developed during the use of oral contraceptives or other estrogen-containing products.

ADVERSE REACTIONS

A variety of major and minor side effects have been attributed to the use of oral contraceptives. Of major concern are cardiovascular side effects and the induction or promotion of tumors. Cigarette smoking increases the risk of serious cardiovascular side effects from oral contraceptives and the risk increases with age and with heavy smoking.

An increased risk of the following serious adverse reactions has been associated with the use of oral contraceptives: thrombophlebitis, pulmonary embolism, coronary thrombosis, cerebral thrombosis, cerebral hemorrhage, hypertension, gallbladder disease, liver tumors, congenital anomalies.

There is evidence of an association between the following conditions and the use of oral contraceptives, although additional confirmatory studies are needed: mesenteric thrombosis, neuro-ocular lesions, e.g., retinal thrombosis and optic neuritis.

The following adverse reactions have been reported in patients receiving oral contraceptives and are believed to be drug-related:

Nausea and/or vomiting, usually the most common adverse reactions, occur in approximately 10% or less of patients during the first cycle. Other reactions, as a general rule, are seen much less frequently or only occasionally: gastro-intestinal symptoms (such as abdominal cramps and bloating), breakthrough bleeding, spotting, change in menstrual flow, dysmenorrhea, amenorrhea during and after treatment, temporary infertility after discontinuance of treatment, edema, chloasma or melasma which may persist, breast changes: tenderness, enlargement, and secretion, change in weight (increase or decrease), change in cervical erosion and cervical secretion, possible diminution in lactation when given immediately postpartum, cholestatic jaundice, migraine, increase in size of uterine leiomyomata, rash (allergic), mental depression, reduced tolerance to carbohydrates, vaginal candidiasis, change in corneal curvature (steepening), intolerance to contact lenses.

The following adverse reactions have been reported in users of oral contraceptives, and the association has been neither confirmed nor refuted: premenstrual-like syndrome, cataracts, changes in libido, chorea, changes in appetite, cystitis-like syndrome, headache, nervousness, dizziness, hirsutism, loss of scalp hair, erythema multiforme, erythema nodosum, hemorrhagic eruption, vaginitis, porphyria, impaired renal function.

The extensive use of oral contraceptives among women throughout the world has prompted many studies aimed at determining toxicity and other effects of these agents. The data have, in some cases, proved to be convincing whereas in others the associations between the drugs and the reactions have been neither confirmed nor refuted. The literature citation below gives a balanced summary and contains further references.

231

LITERATURE   Murad, F, Haynes, RC, Jr: In The Pharma-
              cological Basis of Therapeutics, 6th ed
              (Gilman, AG, Goodman, LS, Gilman, A,
              eds). New York, Macmillan, 1980, Chap-
              ter 61.

OVULEN 21® (Searle)

Ethynodiol diacetate
Mestranol

1981:148
1980:131
1979:113

Ovulen 21 is a combination oral contraceptive preparation. It acts mainly through the mechanism of gonadotropin suppression due to the estrogenic and progestational activity of the constitutents. The predominant effect of estrogen is to inhibit secretion of FSH, while continued action of progesterone (related, but not equated to progestins) is to inhibit LH. Alterations in the genital tract, such as changes in the cervical mucus and the endometrium, may also contribute to the contraceptive effectiveness.

INDICATIONS   For the prevention of pregnancy in women who elect to use oral contraceptives as a method of contraception.

PREPARATIONS   Tablets: ethynodiol diacetate 1 mg and mestranol 0.1 mg.

DOSAGE   1 tablet daily for 21 days according to either of the following schedules: #1 *Sunday Start.* One tablet daily starting on the first Sunday after the onset of menstruation. (If the period begins on Sunday the patient takes her first tablet that same day.) The last (21st) tablet is taken on a Saturday. The next cycle begins on the Sunday, eight days after the last pill of the previous cycle was taken. All subsequent cycles will also begin on Sunday.

#2 *Day 5 Start.* One tablet daily starting on day 5 of her menstrual cycle (the first day of menstruation is counted as day 1) and continues for 21 days. Subsequent cycles begin on the eighth day after taking her last tablet, again starting on the same day of the week on which she began her first course. All subsequent cycles will begin on that same day of the week, that is 1 tablet each day for 3 weeks followed by a week of no pill taking.

CONTRAINDICATIONS AND PRECAUTIONS

Oral contraceptives should not be used in women with any of the following conditions: (1) Thrombophlebitis or thromboembolic disorders. (2) A past history of deep vein thrombophlebitis or thromboembolic disorders. (3) Cerebral vascular or coronary artery disease. (4) Known or suspected carcinoma of the breast. (5) Known or suspected estrogen-dependent neoplasia. (6) Undiagnosed, abnormal genital bleeding. (7) Known or suspected pregnancy. (8) Benign or malignant liver tumor which developed during the use of oral contraceptives or other estrogen-containing products.

ADVERSE REACTIONS

A variety of major and minor side effects have been attributed to the use of oral contraceptives. Of major concern are cardiovascular side effects and the induction or promotion of tumors. Cigarette smoking increases the risk of serious cardiovascular side effects from oral contraceptives and the risk increases with age and with heavy smoking.

An increased risk of the following serious adverse reactions has been associated with the use of oral contraceptives: thrombophlebitis, pulmonary embolism, coronary thrombosis, cerebral thrombosis, cerebral hemorrhage, hypertension, gallbladder disease, liver tumors, congenital anomalies.

There is evidence of an association between the following conditions and the use of oral contraceptives, although additional confirmatory studies are needed: mesenteric thrombosis, neuro-ocular lesions, e.g., retinal thrombosis and optic neuritis.

The following adverse reactions have been reported in patients receiving oral contraceptives and are believed to be drug-related:

Nausea and/or vomiting, usually the most common adverse reactions, occur in approximately 10% or less of patients during the first cycle. Other reactions, as a general rule, are seen much less frequently or only occasionally: gastrointestinal symptoms (such as abdominal cramps and bloating), breakthrough bleeding, spotting, change in menstrual flow, dysmenorrhea, amenorrhea during and after treatment, temporary infertility after discontinuance of treatment, edema, chloasma or melasma which may persist, breast changes: tenderness, enlargement, and secretion, change in weight (increase or decrease), change in cervical erosion and cervical secretion, possible diminution in lactation when given immediately postpartum, cholestatic jaundice, migraine, increase in size of uterine leiomyomata, rash (allergic), mental depression, reduced tolerance to carbohydrates, vaginal candidiasis, change in corneal curvature (steepening), intolerance to contact lenses.

The following adverse reactions have been reported in users of oral contraceptives, and the association has been neither confirmed nor refuted: premenstrual-like syndrome, cataracts, changes in libido, chorea, changes in appetite, cystitis-like syndrome, headache, nervousness, dizziness, hirsutism, loss of scalp hair, erythema multiforme, erythema nodosum, hemorrhagic eruption, vaginitis, porphyria, impaired renal function.

The extensive use of oral contraceptives among women throughout the world has prompted many studies aimed at determining toxicity and other effects of these agents. The data have, in some cases, proved to be convincing whereas in others the associations between the drugs and the reactions have been neither confirmed nor refuted. The literature citation below gives a balanced summary and contains further references.

LITERATURE Murad, F, Haynes, RC, Jr: In The Pharmacological Basis of Therapeutics, 6th ed (Gilman, AG, Goodman, LS, Gilman, A, eds). New York, Macmillan, 1980, Chapter 61.

PARAFON FORTE® (McNeil)
Chlorzoxazone
Acetaminophen

1981:93
1980:78
1979:77

Parafon Forte contains a muscle relaxant and an analgesic and is used to reduce stiffness and limitation of motion associated with many musculoskeletal disorders. Relaxation of skeletal muscle spasm is due to chlorzoxazone, a centrally acting muscle relaxant similar in effect to mephensin. The analgesia is produced by acetaminophen, a nonsalicylate analgesic useful in skeletal muscle pain. Chlorzoxazone acts primarily at the levels of the spinal cord and subcortical areas of the brain, where it inhibits multisynaptic reflex arcs involved in producing and maintaining skeletal muscle spasm of varied etiology.

235

INDICATIONS	Probably effective as an adjunct to rest and physical therapy for relief of discomfort associated with acute, painful musculoskeletal conditions.
PREPARATIONS	Tablets: chlorzoxazone 250 mg and acetaminophen 300 mg.
DOSAGE	Usual adult dosage is 2 tablets four times daily.
CONTRAINDICATIONS AND PRECAUTIONS	Known sensitivity to either components is a contraindication. The safe use in pregnancy or in nursing mothers has not been established. Caution should be observed in patients with a history of allergies to drugs. The concomitant use of alcohol or other CNS depressants may have an additive effect. This drug should be discontinued if signs of liver dysfunction appear.
ADVERSE REACTIONS	Chlorzoxazone has been used in an estimated 23 million patients and is apparently well tolerated. Occasionally gastrointestinal disturbances, and sensitivity reactions develop. Drowsiness and other CNS effects are very rare; other reactions such as angioneurotic edema, anaphylactic reactions or liver dysfunction are extremely rare. Acetaminophen side effects are uncommon. Among 1215 patients receiving acetaminophen observed in the Boston Collaborative Drug Surveillance Program 4 patients had adverse reactions as follows: diaphoresis (2), gastrointestinal disturbances (1), and sensitivity reaction (1).
LITERATURE	Gready, DM: Curr Ther Res 20:666, 1976; Walker, JM: Curr Ther Res 15:249, 1973. For a discussion of the pharmacology of spasticity see Davidoff, RA: Neurology (Minneapolis) 28:46, 1978.

PAVABID® (Marion)
Papaverine HCl

1981:124
1980:100
1979: 82

Papaverine is a nonspecific smooth muscle relaxant capable of dilat-
ing arteries in the coronary, cerebral, and systemic circulations. It
also has been shown to depress A-V nodal and intraventricular conduction in high enough doses. Though widely prescribed in the
treatment of cerebral spasm and myocardial ischemia complicated
by arrhythmias, its efficacy in these conditions is questionable.

INDICATIONS	For the relief of cerebral and peripheral ischemia associated with arterial spasm and myocardial ischemia complicated by arrhythmias.
PREPARATIONS	Capsules: 150 and 300 mg.
DOSAGE	One 150 mg capsule every 12 hours. In difficult cases the dosage is one 300 mg capsule every 8–12 hours.
CONTRAINDICATIONS AND PRECAUTIONS	Use cautiously in patients with glaucoma. Discontinue this medication if hepatic hypersensitivity develops.
ADVERSE REACTIONS	Reported side effects, though rare, include gastrointestinal disturbances, malaise, drowsiness, vertigo, sweating, headache, and skin rash. Among 203 patients on papaverine HCl studied in the Boston Collaborative Drug Surveillance Program 5 patients had adverse effects as follows: hypotension, vertigo, or headache (4), palpitations (1).
LITERATURE	Branconnier, RJ, Cole, J: J Am Geriatr Soc 25:458, 1977; Culebras: A: Neurology 26:673, 1976; FDA Drug Bull 9:26, 1979; Medical Letter 23:37, 1981; Ritter, RM, et al: J Contin Educ Clin Med 18:18,20, 1971.

PENICILLIN V Potassium

1981:11
1980:11
1979:14

Penicillin V, the phenoxymethyl analogue of penicillin G, is a semi-synthetic penicillin for *oral* use; discussed here is the potassium salt of penicillin V (often called Penicillin VK). This drug is more stable in acid than is penicillin G and, thus, it is better absorbed from the gastrointestinal tract. Its actions are the same as those of penicillin G for gram-positive microorganisms and it is, therefore, preferable to penicillin G in cases in which the oral route is desirable, but it is less effective than penicillin G against gram-negative microorganisms, especially *Neisseria* species. (Thus, it is not recommended for gonococcal infections.) Like penicillin G, this agent is not effective against penicillinase-producing bacteria.

INDICATIONS

Penicillin V potassium is indicated in the treatment of mild to moderately severe infections due to penicillin G-sensitive microorganisms. This drug is indicated for mild to moderate streptococcal infections of the upper respiratory tract, scarlet fever, and mild erysipelas; mild to moderate pneumococcal infections of the respiratory tract; mild penicillin G-sensitive staphylococcal infections of the skin and soft tissues. (Reports indicate an increasing number of resistant strains.) Infections of the oropharynx, mild to moderate, due to *Fusospirochetes* (Vincent's gingivitis and pharyngitis) usually respond. It is indicated for the prevention of recurrence following rheumatic fever and/or chorea and for prevention of infections in certain cardiac patients undergoing dental procedures or minor upper respiratory tract surgery or instrumentation. Prophylaxis should be started on the day of the procedure and continued for 2 or more days following.

PREPARATIONS

Tablets: 125, 250, and 500 mg. Powder for oral solution; 125 and 250 mg/5 ml. (See also PEN-VEE-K and V-CILLIN K)

DOSAGE

The usual adult oral dosage range is 125–500 mg four to six times daily. The usual oral dosage range in children is 25–50 mg/kg body weight daily administered in divided doses every 6–8 hours. For prophylactic treatment of rheumatic fever in adults, 125–250 mg daily.

CONTRAINDICATIONS AND PRECAUTIONS

Known hypersensitivity to penicillins is a contraindication; use cautiously in patients with allergies and/or asthma.

ADVERSE REACTIONS

Hypersensitivity reactions are fairly common (1 to 5%), gastrointestinal reactions occur, and superinfections with resistant organisms (such as gram-negative bacteria) can occur. Blood dyscrasias, neuropathy, and nephropathy occur rarely and are usually associated with high doses of parenteral penicillin. The penicillins are otherwise essentially nontoxic in man. Among 707 patients on penicillin VK studied in the Boston Collaborative Drug Surveillance Program 19 patients had side effects as follows: sensitivity reactions (10), gastrointestinal disturbances (6), and "other" (3).

LITERATURE

AMA Drug Evaluations, 4th ed. New York, AMA and Wiley, 1980, Chapter 69; Mandell, GL, Sande, MA: In The Pharmacological Basis of Therapeutics, 6th ed (Gilman, AG, Goodman, LS, Gilman, A, eds). New York, Macmillan, 1980, Chapter 50; Medical Letter 24:21, 1982 (choice of antimicrobials).

Penicillin V, the phenoxymethyl analogue of penicillin G, is a semi-synthetic penicillin for *oral* use; discussed here is the potassium salt of penicillin V (often called Penicillin VK). This drug is more stable in acid than is penicillin G and, thus, it is better absorbed from the gastrointestinal tract. Its actions are the same as those of penicillin G for gram-positive microorganisms and it is, therefore, preferable to penicillin G in cases in which the oral route is desirable, but it is less effective than penicillin G against gram-negative microorganisms, especially *Neisseria* species. (Thus, it is not recommended for gonococcal infections.) Like penicillin G, this agent is not effective against penicillinase-producing bacteria.

INDICATIONS

Penicillin V potassium is indicated in the treatment of mild to moderately severe infections due to penicillin G-sensitive microorganisms. This drug is indicated for mild to moderate streptococcal infections of the upper respiratory tract, scarlet fever, and mild erysipelas; mild to moderate pneumococcal infections of the respiratory tract; mild penicillin G-sensitive staphylococcal infections of the skin and soft tissues. (Reports indicate an increasing number of resistant strains.) Infections of the oropharynx, mild to moderate, due to *Fusospirochetes* (Vincent's gingivitis and pharyngitis) usually respond. It is indicated for the prevention of recurrence following rheumatic fever and/or chorea and for prevention of infections in certain cardiac patients undergoing dental procedures or minor upper respiratory tract surgery or instrumentation. Prophylaxis should be started on the day of the procedure and continued for 2 or more days following.

PREPARATIONS

Tablets: 125, 250, and 500 mg. Powder for oral solution: 125 and 250 mg/5 ml.

DOSAGE

The usual adult oral dosage range is 125–500 mg four to six times daily. The usual oral dosage range in children is 25–50 mg/kg body weight daily administered in divided doses every 6–8 hours. For prophylactic treatment of rheumatic fever in adults, 125–250 mg daily.

CONTRAINDICATIONS AND PRECAUTIONS

Known hypersensitivity to penicillins is a contraindication; use cautiously in patients with allergies and/or asthma.

ADVERSE REACTIONS

Hypersensitivity reactions are fairly common (1 to 5%), gastrointestinal reactions occur, and superinfections with resistant organisms (such as gram-negative bacteria) can occur. Blood dyscrasias, neuropathy, and nephropathy occur rarely and are usually associated with high doses of parenteral penicillin. The penicillins are otherwise essentially nontoxic in man. Among 707 patients on penicillin VK studied in the Boston Collaborative Drug Surveillance Program 19 patients had side effects as follows: sensitivity reactions (10), gastrointestinal disturbances (6), and "other" (3).

LITERATURE

AMA Drug Evaluations, 4th ed. New York, AMA and Wiley, 1980, Chapter 69; Mandell, GL, Sande, MA: In The Pharmacological Basis of Therapeutics, 6th ed (Gilman, AG, Goodman, LS, Gilman, A, eds). New York, Macmillan, 1980, Chapter 50; Medical Letter, 24:21, 1982 (choice of antimicrobials).

PERCODAN® (Endo)

Oxycodone HCl
Oxycodone terephthalate
Aspirin

1981:73
1980:56
1979:50

The principal ingredient, oxycodone, is a semisynthetic narcotic analgesic with multiple actions qualitatively similar to those of morphine. The most prominent of these involve the central nervous system and organs composed of smooth muscle. The principal actions of therapeutic value of the oxycodone in Percodan are analgesia and sedation. Oxycodone is similar to codeine and methadone in that it retains one half its analgesic activity when administered orally.

INDICATIONS	For the relief of moderate to moderately severe pain.
PREPARATIONS	Tablets: oxycodone hydrochloride 4.50 mg, oxycodone terephthalate 0.38 mg and aspirin 325 mg.
DOSAGE	The usual adult dose is 1 tablet every 6 hours as needed for pain. The dosage should be adjusted according to the severity of the pain.
CONTRAINDICATIONS AND PRECAUTIONS	Hypersensitivity to any of the ingredients of Percodan is a contraindication. This preparation should be used cautiously by pregnant women, children, in patients using other CNS depressants and in patients who require complete mental alertness (because Percodan may impair mental and/or physical abilities). Caution should also be used in patients with head injury, acute abdominal conditions and in special risk patients (such as those with renal and/or hepatic disease or the elderly).

ADVERSE REACTIONS   Gastrointestinal disturbances, light-head-edness, and other CNS effects are the most common adverse reactions. Other adverse reactions include dry mouth, euphoria, dysphoria, and pruritis. Oxycodone can produce drug dependence of the morphine type. Among 423 patients on Percodan in the Boston Collaborative Drug Surveillance Program 19 patients had adverse reactions as follows: gastrointestinal disturbances (9), CNS effects (7), dry mouth (1), gastrointestinal bleeding (1), rise in serum amylase level (1).

The CNS depressant effects of Percodan can be addictive with those of other CNS depressants. Aspirin can enhance the effects of anticoagulants and inhibit the effects of uricosuric agents.

LITERATURE   AMA Drug Evaluations, 4th ed. New York, AMA and Wiley, 1980, p 83. For additional information on pain relievers, see Beaver, WT: Analgesic combinations. In Combination Drugs: Their Use and Regulation (Lasagna, L, ed). New York, Stratton Intercontinental, 1975.

PERIACTIN® (Merck Sharp & Dohme)
Cyproheptadine HCl

1981:146
1980:145
1979:130

Periactin is a serotonin and histamine (H_1) antagonist with anticholinergic and sedative effects.

INDICATIONS   Periactin is indicated in perennial and seasonal rhinitis, vasomotor rhinitis, allergic conjunctivitis due to inhalant allergens

243

and foods, and in mild, uncomplicated skin manifestations of urticaria and angioedema. It is indicated in the amelioration of allergic reactions to blood or plasma, in the treatment of cold urticaria, and in dermatographism. The serotonin-blocking property of cyproheptadine is useful in treating the postgastrectomy dumping syndrome, intestinal hypermotility of carcinoid, and some other conditions involving the release of serotonin.

PREPARATIONS

Tablets: 4 mg. Syrup: concentration 2 mg per 5 ml (teaspoon).

DOSAGE

The dosage is individualized. Adults: 4–20 mg/day. This dosage should be started as 4 mg three times a day and then adjusted. Children, age 2–6 years: 2 mg two or three times daily; age 7–14 years: 4 mg two or three times daily. The dosage in small children may be computed on the basis of body weight, 0.25 mg/kg daily.

CONTRAINDICATIONS AND PRECAUTIONS

Periactin should not be used in newborn or premature infants, nursing mothers, or elderly, debilitated patients. Antihistamines should not be used to treat lower respiratory tract symptoms including asthma. Periactin should not be used by patients with any of the following conditions: angle-closure glaucoma, stenosing peptic ulcer, symptomatic prostatic hypertrophy, bladder-neck obstruction, pyloroduodenal obstruction, or hypersensitivity to cyproheptadine. Antihistamines should be used with caution in children, pregnant women, and patients receiving CNS depressants concomitantly.

ADVERSE REACTIONS

Drowsiness is the most common adverse reaction. Dryness of mouth, nose, and throat, thickening of bronchial secretions, dizziness, epigastric distress, and disturbed coordination may occur with antihistamines. (See package insert for further details on adverse reactions.)

It is noteworthy that MAO inhibitors prolong and intensify the anticholinergic effects of antihistamines.

LITERATURE

AMA Drug Evaluations, 4th ed. New York, AMA and Wiley, 1980, Chapter 28; Jilhewar, AG, Collins, DM: Ir Med J 70(2):50, 1977; (case report on cold urticaria); Kuokkamen, K: Acta Allergol 32:316, 1977 (chronic urticaria); Sigler, RW, et al: J Allergy Clin Immunol 63(3):173, 1979 (cold urticaria).

PERSANTINE® (Boehringer Ingelheim)
Dipyridamole

1981:62
1980:69
1979:81

Dipyridamole, a coronary vasodilator, is unrelated chemically to the nitrates or digitalis. In therapeutic doses this drug usually produces no significant alteration of systemic blood flow in peripheral arteries. It increases coronary artery blood flow primarily by a selective dilation of the coronary arteries, but evidence for its efficacy in treating angina pectoris is questionable.

INDICATIONS

Persantine may be useful in the long-term therapy of chronic angina pectoris. Prolonged therapy may reduce the frequency or eliminate anginal episodes, improve exercise tolerance, and reduce nitroglycerin requirements. The drug is not intended to abort the acute anginal attack.

PREPARATIONS

Tablets: 25, 50, and 75 mg.

245

DOSAGE

The recommended dosage is 50 mg three times a day, taken at least 1 hour before meals.

CONTRAINDICATIONS AND PRECAUTIONS

No specific contraindications are known. The 25 mg tablet contains FD C #5 (tartrazine) which cross-reacts with patients with aspirin sensitivity. Hence, caution should be used when this tablet (25 mg) is used in patients with aspirin sensitivity.

ADVERSE REACTIONS

Dizziness, headache, syncope, gastrointestinal disturbances, and rash. Although rare, this drug has appeared to aggravate anginal symptoms. Dipyridamole is known to increase or normalize shortened platelet survival and aspirin may potentiate this effect in a dose-related fashion (Moncada and Korbut, 1978).

LITERATURE

Coeugniet, E: Thromb Res 7(1):251, 1975; Damasio, H: Lancet 2(8087):478, 1978 (migraine); Fassio, G, et al: J Int Med Res 7:492, 1979 (aspirin plus dipyridamole in transient ischemia); Genton, E, et al: N Engl J Med 293:1174, 1236, and 1296, 1975 (platelet-inhibiting drugs and thrombotic disease). Moncada, S, Korbut, R, Lancet, June 17, 1978, p 1286.

PHENAPHEN® /CODEINE (Robins)
Acetaminophen
Codeine phosphate

1981:112
1980: 91
1979: 79

Acetaminophen is a nonsalicylate analgesic and antipyretic. Codeine is an analgesic and antitussive.

INDICATIONS

Phenaphen with codeine No. 2 and Phenaphen with codeine No. 3 are indicated for the relief of mild to moderate pain. Phenaphen with codeine No. 4 is indicated for the relief of moderate to severe pain. Phenaphen-650 with codeine is indicated for the relief of mild to moderate pain.

PREPARATIONS

Capsules: Nos. 2, 3, and 4 each containing acetaminophen 325 mg and codeine phosphate 15, 30, and 60 mg, respectively. Also available as Phenaphen-650 with codeine in which each tablet contains acetaminophen 650 mg plus codeine phosphate 30 mg.

DOSAGE

Though dosage should be individualized, the usual adult dose for Nos. 2 and 3 capsules is 1 or 2 capsules every 4 hours as required. The usual dose for No. 4 capsules and Phenaphen-650/codeine is 1 every 4 hours as required.

CONTRAINDICATIONS AND PRECAUTIONS

Phenaphen/codeine should not be used by patients with hypersensitivity to codeine or acetaminophen. Codeine and acetaminophen should be used with caution in pregnant women and patients receiving CNS depressants concomitantly.

ADVERSE REACTIONS

The most frequently reported side effects include lightheadedness, dizziness, sedation, nausea, and vomiting. Other reactions are euphoria, dysphoria, constipation, and pruritis. Codeine may be habit forming. Acetaminophen effects were observed in 1215 patients studied in the Boston Collaborative Drug Surveillance Program and 4 adverse reactions occurred: diaphoresis (2), gastrointestinal disturbances (1), and sensitivity reactions (1). The CNS depressant action of these preparations may be additive with those of other CNS depressants.

247

LITERATURE The actions of codeine are well known. The pharmacology and toxicity of acetaminophen is contained in the reviews by Ameer and Greenblatt: Ann Int Med 87:202, 1977, and Koch-Weser: N Eng J Med 295(23):1297, 1976.

PHENERGAN® EXPECTORANT (Wyeth)

Promethazine HCl
Guaiacolsulfonate potassium
Sodium citrate
Citric acid anhydrous
Ipecac fluid extract
Alcohol

This combination of ingredients preparation is intended to aid in the treatment of coughs due to colds, allergies, and minor upper respiratory disorders. The promethazine component possesses sedative, antihistaminic, and antiemetic actions. Guaiacolsulfonate is possibly effective in increasing respiratory tract secretions.

INDICATIONS Coughs due to colds, allergies, and minor upper respiratory disorders.

PREPARATIONS Liquid: each 5 ml contains promethazine HCl 5 mg, guaiacolsulfonate potassium 44 mg, sodium citrate 197 mg, citric acid anhydrous 60 mg, ipecac fluid extract 0.17 min, and alcohol 7%.

DOSAGE Usual adult dosage is 1 teaspoon (5 ml) every 4–6 hours as needed, for patients confined to home. Ambulatory, fully active patients should be checked to guard against drowsiness with this preparation.

CONTRAINDICATIONS AND PRECAUTIONS	Alcohol and other CNS depressants should not be used when on this preparation.
ADVERSE REACTIONS	Drowsiness can occur. Occasionally, autonomic reactions occur such as dryness of mouth, blurred vision and, rarely, dizziness. Very rare cases of leukopenia and one case of agranulocytosis have been reported in patients receiving promethazine, usually in association with other agents known to cause these conditions. Hyperexcitability and nightmares have occurred in children receiving large oral doses of promethazine. Interactions may occur with concomitant use of amphetamines, anticholinergics, levodopa, antacids, and trihexyphenidyl. Promethazine hydrochloride, in *much higher* doses than that in this preparation, and given by alternate routes for different situations, was studied in 826 patients in the Boston Collaborative Drug Surveillance Program. Twenty-seven patients had side effects as follows: drowsiness and confusion (19), CNS excitation (3), hypotension (2), respiratory depression (1), dry mouth (1), and injection site complications (1).
LITERATURE	For a comprehensive review on cough, see Irwin, RS, et al: Arch Intern Med 137:1186, 1977.

PHENERGAN® EXPECTORANT/Codeine
(Wyeth)
Promethazine HCl
Guaiacolsulfonate potassium
Sodium citrate
Citric acid anhydrous
Ipecac fluid extract
Alcohol
Codeine phosphate

1981:75
1980:70
1979:71

This combination of ingredients preparation is intended to aid in the treatment of coughs due to colds, allergies, and minor upper respiratory disorders. The promethazine component possesses sedative, antihistaminic, and antiemetic actions. Guaiacolsulfonate is possibly effective in increasing respiratory tract secretions. Codeine is an antitussive.

INDICATIONS	Coughs due to colds, allergies, and minor upper respiratory disorders.
PREPARATIONS	Liquid: each 5 ml contains promethazine HCl 5 mg, guaiacolsulfonate potassium 44 mg, sodium citrate 197 mg, citric acid anhydrous 60 mg, ipecac fluid extract 0.17 min, alcohol 7%, and codeine phosphate 10 mg.
DOSAGE	Usual adult dosage is 1 teaspoon (5 ml) every 4–6 hours as needed, for patients confined to home. Ambulatory, fully active patients should be checked to guard against drowsiness with this preparation.
CONTRAINDICATIONS AND PRECAUTIONS	Alcohol and other CNS depressants should not be used when on this preparation.
ADVERSE REACTIONS	Drowsiness can occur. Occasionally, autonomic reactions occur such as dryness of

mouth, blurred vision and, rarely, dizziness. Very rare cases of leukopenia and one case of agranulocytosis have been reported in patients receiving promethazine, usually in association with other agents known to cause these conditions. Hyperexcitability and nightmares have occurred in children receiving large oral doses of promethazine. Interactions may occur with concomitant use of amphetamines, anticholinergics, levodopa, antacids, and trihexyphenidyl. Promethazine hydrochloride, in *much higher* doses than that in this preparation, and given by alternate routes for different situations, was studied in 826 patients in the Boston Collaborative Drug Surveillance Program. Twenty-seven patients had side effects as follows: drowsiness and confusion (19), CNS excitation (3), hypotension (2), respiratory depression (1), dry mouth (1), and injection site complications (1).

LITERATURE   For a comprehensive review on cough, see Irwin, RS, et al: Arch Intern Med 137:1186, 1977.

PHENERGAN® VC EXPECTORANT (Wyeth)   1981:182
Promethazine HCl   1980:167
Guaiacolsulfonate potassium   1979:166
Sodium citrate
Citric acid
Ipecac fluid extract
Alcohol
Phenylephrine HCl

This combination of ingredients preparation is intended to aid in the treatment of coughs due to colds, allergies, and minor upper respiratory disorders. The promethazine component possesses sedative, antihistaminic, and antiemetic actions. Guaiacolsulfonate is possibly effective in increasing respiratory tract secretions.

INDICATIONS

Coughs due to colds, allergies, and minor upper respiratory disorders.

PREPARATIONS

Liquid: each 5 ml contains promethazine HCl 5 mg, guaiacolsulfonate potassium 44 mg, sodium citrate 197 mg, citric acid anhydrous 60 mg, ipecac fluid extract 0.17 min, alcohol 7%, and phenylephrine HCl 5 mg.

DOSAGE

Usual adult dosage is 1 teaspoon (5 ml) every 4–6 hours as needed, for patients confined to home. Ambulatory, fully active patients should be checked to guard against drowsiness with this preparation.

CONTRAINDICATIONS AND PRECAUTIONS

Use cautiously in patients with diabetes, hyperthyroidism, or cardiovascular disease. Alcohol and other CNS depressants should not be used while on this preparation.

ADVERSE REACTIONS

Drowsiness can occur. Occasionally, autonomic reactions occur such as dryness of the mouth, blurred vision and, rarely, dizziness. Very rare cases of leukopenia and one case of agranulocytosis have been reported in patients receiving promethazine, usually in association with other agents known to cause these conditions. Hyperexcitability and nightmares have occurred in children receiving large oral doses of promethazine. Interactions may occur with concomitant use of amphetamines, anticholinergics, levodopa, antacids, trihexphenidyl, guanethidine, MAO inhibitors, and antidepressants. Promethazine hydrochloride, in *much higher* doses than that in this preparation, and given by alternate routes for different situations, was studied in 826 patients in the Boston Collaborative Drug Surveillance Program. Twenty-seven patients had side effects as follows: drowsiness and confusion (19), CNS excitation (3), hypotension (2), respiratory depression (1), dry mouth (1), and injection site complications (1).

LITERATURE   For a comprehensive review on cough, see Irwin, RS, et al: Arch Intern Med 137:1186, 1977.

PHENERGAN® VC EXPECTORANT/CODEINE   1981:111
(Wyeth)   1980: 96
Promethazine HCl   1979:102
Guaiacolsulfonate potassium
Sodium citrate
Citric acid
Ipecac fluid extract
Alcohol
Phenylephrine HCl
Codeine phosphate

This combination of ingredients preparation is intended to aid in the treatment of coughs due to colds, allergies, and minor upper respiratory disorders. The promethazine component possesses sedative, antihistaminic, and antiemetic actions. Guaiacolsulfonate is possibly effective in increasing respiratory tract secretions. Codeine is an antitussive.

INDICATIONS   Coughs due to colds, allergies, and minor upper respiratory disorders.

PREPARATIONS   Liquid: each 5 ml contains promethazine

HCl 5 mg, guaiacolsulfonate potassium 44 mg, sodium citrate 197 mg, citric acid anhydrous 60 mg, ipecac fluid extract 0.17 min, alcohol 7%, phenylephrine HCl 5 mg, and codeine phosphate 10 mg.

DOSAGE

Usual adult dosage is 1 teaspoon (5 ml) every 4–6 hours as needed, for patients confined to home. Ambulatory, fully active, patients should be checked to guard against drowsiness with this preparation.

CONTRAINDICATIONS AND PRECAUTIONS

Use cautiously in patients with diabetes, hyperthyroidism, cardiovascular disease and in addiction-prone patients. Alcohol and other CNS depressants should not be used while on this preparation.

ADVERSE REACTIONS

Drowsiness can occur. Occasionally, autonomic reactions occur such as dryness of the mouth, blurred vision and, rarely, dizziness. Very rare cases of leukopenia and one case of agranulocytosis have been reported in patients receiving promethazine, usually in association with other agents known to cause these conditions. Hyperexcitability and nightmares have occurred in children receiving large oral doses of promethazine. Interactions may occur with concomitant use of amphetamines, anticholinergics, levodopa, antacids, trihexyphenidyl, guanethidine, MAO inhibitors, and antidepressants. Promethazine hydrochloride, in *much higher* doses than that in this preparation, and given by alternate routes for different situations, was studied in 826 patients in the Boston Collaborative Drug Surveillance Program. Twenty-seven patients had side effects as follows: drowsiness and confusion (19), CNS excitation (3), hypotension (2), respiratory depression (1), dry mouth (1), and injection site complications (1).

LITERATURE   For a comprehensive review on cough, see Irwin, RS, et al: Arch Intern Med 137:1186, 1977.

PHENOBARBITAL

1981:39
1980:40
1979:38

Phenobarbital has effects on nervous tissue. It depresses the central nervous system, producing in small doses a sedative effect, and in larger doses a state called hypnosis that resembles nocturnal sleep. It has anticonvulsant and antiepileptic properties. One of the best-known barbiturates, phenobarbital is classed as long-acting because of its slow rate of absorption from the gastrointestinal tract and its slow rate of metabolism. Its rate of entry into the central nervous system is slow compared to other barbiturates. It is generally believed that barbiturates are not significantly analgesic. Like other barbiturates, phenobarbital depresses respiration and has autonomic effects that appear at high doses but are usually slight at ordinary hypnotic doses.

INDICATIONS   Sedation and hypnosis; management of grand mal epilepsy.

PREPARATIONS   Elixir: 20 mg/5ml. Tablets: 7.5, 15, 30, 60, 90, and 100 mg. Capsules (timed-release): 60 mg. Parenteral and rectal forms available.

DOSAGE   For sedation in adults: 30–120 mg daily in two or three divided doses; for children 6 mg/kg body weight daily in three divided doses. For hypnosis in adults: 100–320 mg. The hypnotic dose in children must be individualized. The anticonvulsant dose in adults is 50–100 mg two or three times daily; in children 3 to 5 mg per kg of body weight daily. (Consult

255

other sources for use of parenteral forms and rectal forms.)

CONTRAINDICATIONS AND PRECAUTIONS

Porphyria, severe renal or hepatic disease, and pulmonary insufficiency are contraindications, as is barbiturate hypersensitivity.

ADVERSE REACTIONS

Drowsiness is common, though some patients experience CNS excitation (especially children and elderly patients); rashes and gastrointestinal disturbances may occur. Among 1349 patients on phenobarbital studied in the Boston Collaborative Drug Surveillance Program 114 patients had adverse reactions as follows: CNS effects, drowsiness (75), disorientation or confusion (8), excitation, anxiety, agitation, or insomnia (4), coma (2), respiratory depression (2), headache (1), nightmare (1), psychiatric disturbances (3), sensitivity reaction, rash or pruritis (12), drug fever (1), gastrointestinal disturbances (4), and injection site complications (1).

Phenobarbital induces hepatic microsomal enzymes and thus can influence the biotransformation of many drugs (eg, oral anticoagulants, chlorpromazine (see Medical Letter reference). It also has abuse potential. Tolerance also develops to barbiturates.

LITERATURE

Harvey, SC: In The Pharmacological Basis of Therapeutics, 6th ed (Gilman, AG, Goodman, LS, Gilman, A, eds). New York, Macmillan, 1980, Chapter 17 (hypnotics and sedatives); Medical Letter 21:25, 1979 (drugs for epilepsy); Symposium: Antiepileptic Drugs (Woodbury, DM, Penry, JK, Schmidt, RP, eds). New York, Raven Press, 1972.

POLY-VI-FLOR® CHEWABLE (Mead Johnson)

1981:126
1980:116
1979:139

Poly-Vi-Flor chewable tablets contain 10 vitamins plus fluoride for diet supplementation and dental caries prophylaxis.

INDICATIONS	Vitamin supplementation and prevention of caries in children over 3 years of age in areas where the water fluoride level is less than 0.3 ppm.
PREPARATIONS	Tablets (chewable): Vitamins A (2500 IU), D (400 IU), E (15 IU), C (60 mg), folic acid (0.3 mg), B_1 (1.05 mg), B_2 (1.2 mg), niacin (13.5 mg), B_6 (1.05 mg), B_{12} (4.5 μg), and fluoride either 1.0 mg or 0.5 mg (2 strengths available). Also available with iron, 12 mg.
DOSAGE	1 tablet daily for children over 3 years of age.
CONTRAINDICATIONS AND PRECAUTIONS	Not for use in children who regularly consume drinking water with a fluoride content greater than 0.3 ppm or by patients with dental fluorosis.
ADVERSE REACTIONS	Allergic rash occurs rarely.
LITERATURE	Committee on Nutrition, Am Acad Pediatrics: Pediatrics 63:150, 1979; Hennon, DK, et al: J Pediatrics 80:1018, 1972.

POTASSIUM CHLORIDE

Potassium is the predominant intracellular cation. Potassium chloride is used in certain situations in which potassium supplementation is needed.

INDICATIONS
To treat muscular weakness associated with hypokalemia. It is used to counteract the potassium-wasting effect of thiazide and loop diuretics and in treatment programs for diabetic ketoacidosis that may be *expected* to produce acute and severe hypokalemia. Potassium replacement is also indicated in cases of metabolic alkalosis that persist because of an inappropriate excretion of an acidic urine. Additional indications may include situations of inadequate dietary intake of potassium, excessive gastrointestinal losses, potassium-wasting nephropathy, primary adrenal disease, or in patients receiving corticosteroids. Potassium chloride is also used to treat digitalis intoxication.

PREPARATIONS
Liquid: 5, 10, and 20%. (See also SLOW-K and K-LYTE.) Potassium chloride oral solution USP: 20 mEq potassium/15 ml (tablespoon).

DOSAGE
The usual adult oral dose is 10–15 mEq three or four times daily (diluted in ½ glass of cold water or juice). Patients on diuretics may require 80–100 mEq daily.

CONTRAINDICATIONS AND PRECAUTIONS
Potassium supplements are contraindicated in patients receiving potassium-sparing diuretics; use very cautiously in patients with impaired renal function.

Hyperkalemia and associated cardiac toxicity may occur. Gastrointestinal irritation and ulceration are also seen. Among 6797 patients on oral and parenteral potassium chloride studied in the Boston Collaborative Drug Surveillance Program 410 patients had adverse reactions as follows: hyperkalemia (259), gastrointestinal disturbances (109), injection site complications, phlebitis (32), arrhythmias (3), pain (2), hematemesis (1), and "other" (4).

LITERATURE

deWardener, HE, et al: Br Med J 4:168, 1969 (potassium supplements); Lawson, DH: Q J Med 43:433, 1974 (adverse reactions to potassium chloride); McMahon, FG: Management of Essential Hypertension, Mt. Kisco, New York, Futura Publishing, 1978, Chapter 4 (potassium supplements).

PREDNISONE

1981:33
1980:31
1979:30

Prednisone, a synthetic glucocorticoid for oral use, has a powerful anti-inflammatory action in disorders of many organ systems. Glucocorticoids such as prednisone cause a variety of metabolic effects and, in addition, modify the patient's immune response to many different stimuli. Prednisone causes less sodium retention than cortisol and has a somewhat greater anti-inflammatory potency. Corticosteroids may mask signs of infection.

INDICATIONS

For acute use in rheumatic disorders and collagen disease, and for dermatologic diseases; in the treatment of endocrine disorders such as adrenocortical insufficiency (hydrocortisone or cortisone is the first choice) and as adjunctive therapy in other endocrine disorders. Prednisone may be useful in the control of severe allergic conditions intractable to conventional treatment. It is useful in treating severe allergic and inflammatory processes involving the eye and its adnexa. Prednisone and other corticosteroids have a variety of other uses, either alone or in combination with other therapies. These include respiratory disorders, hematologic disorders, and neoplastic disease.

PREPARATIONS

Tablets: 1, 2.5, 5, 10, and 20 mg.

DOSAGE

For rheumatic disorders in adults the initial dose is 4–5 mg daily, gradually (3–7 day intervals) adjusted to a maintenance level not to exceed 10 mg daily; in children 0.4–1.0 mg/kg body weight daily. For inflammatory and allergic conditions the range in *initially* 5–60 mg. For replacement therapy, 5–7.5 mg daily in divided doses (largest dose on arising). When this medication is to be discontinued the dosage should be reduced gradually. (The pediatric dose is governed more by the severity of the condition and the response of the patient than by age or body weight.)

CONTRAINDICATIONS AND PRECAUTIONS

Prednisone should not be used in patients with systemic fungal infections. Corticosteroids should be used with extreme caution in pregnant women and nursing mothers. Vaccination and other immunization procedures should not be undertaken while a patient is on corticosteroid therapy. Patients with latent tuberculosis or tuberculin reactivity should be closely monitored for reactivation. Use cautiously when the following conditions exist: cardiac disease, diabetes mellitus, myasthenia gravis, peptic ulcer, gastritis, or esophagitis.

ADVERSE REACTIONS

Acute adrenal insufficiency may result from too rapid withdrawal of corticosteroids after prolonged therapy. Other side effects, resulting from prolonged therapy are fluid and electrolyte imbalance, hyperglycemia and glycosuria, increased susceptibility to infections, peptic ulcers, behavioral disturbances, Cushing's syndrome, arrest of growth, and other disturbances. Among 1793 patients on prednisone studied in the Boston Collaborative Drug Surveillance Program 270 patients had adverse reactions as follows: fluid or electrolyte disorders (45), Cushing's syndrome (40), gastrointestinal bleeding (40), psychiatric disturbances (38), hyperglycemia (36), gastrointestinal disturbances other than bleeding (34), and "other" (37). Corticosteroids interact with barbiturates, potassium-wasting diuretics, ephedrine, phenytoin, rifampin, and curare. It is noteworthy that steroids can mask the signs and symptoms of inflammation and many disease processes.

LITERATURE

Azarnoff, DL, ed: Steroid Therapy. Philadelphia, Saunders 1975; Ehrlich, GE: Mod Med 46:78, 1978 (steroids in rheumatic disease).

PREMARIN® (Ayerst)
Conjugated estrogens

1981:24
1980:25
1979:25

Premarin contains a mixture of estrogens obtained from natural sources. These consist of estrone, equilin and 17-alpha-dihydroequilin together with smaller amounts of 17-alpha-estrodiol, equilenin, and 17-alpha-dihydroequilenin. Estrogens are important in the development and maintenance of the female reproductive system and secondary sex characteristics. The pharmacologic effects of conjugated estrogens are similar to those of endogenous estrogens.

INDICATIONS

Premarin is indicated for moderate to severe vasomotor symptoms associated with menopause, atrophic vaginitis, kraurosis vulvae, female hypogonadism, female castration, primary ovarian failure, and as palliative treatment for breast cancer and prostatic carcinoma. It is also used for postpartum breast engorgement. Premarin is not effective for any purpose during pregnancy.

PREPARATIONS

Tablets: 0.3, 0.625, 1.25, and 2.5 mg.

DOSAGE

Cyclic usage for short-term, as in treating vasomotor symptoms, 1.25 mg daily (if patient is menstruating, start on day 5); in treating atrophic vaginitis and kraurosis vulvae, 0.3–1.25 mg daily. For treating female hypogonadism, 2.5–7.5 mg daily, in divided doses for 20 days, followed by no therapy for 10 days. If bleeding does not occur by the end of this time, the same dosage schedule is repeated. If bleeding occurs before the end of the 10 day period, begin a 20 day estrogen-progestin cyclic regimen with 2.5–7.5 mg of Premarin daily, in divided doses for 20 days. During the last 5 days of estrogen therapy an oral progestin is given. If bleeding occurs before this regimen is concluded, therapy is discontinued and may be resumed on the 5th day of bleeding.

In female castration and primary ovarian failure, 1.25 mg daily, cyclically (adjust to lowest level needed for maintenance). For inoperable progressing breast cancer, in appropriately selected men and postmenopausal women, 10 mg three times daily for at least 3 months. For osteoporosis, 1.25 mg daily, cyclically. For inoperable progressing prostatic cancer, Premarin is used chronically, 1.25–2.5 mg three times daily.

CONTRAINDICATIONS AND PRECAUTIONS

Estrogens should not be used by persons with any of the following conditions: known or suspected pregnancy, known or suspected cancer of the breast except in certain selected patients with metastatic disease, known or suspected estrogen dependent neoplasia, undiagnosed abnormal genital bleeding, active thromboembolic disorders, or a history of thromboembolic disorders with estrogen use. Premarin should be used with caution in patients with high blood pressure or diabetes.

ADVERSE REACTIONS

Nausea is the most frequent adverse effect of estrogens. Estrogens have been reported to increase the risk of endometrial carcinoma; they may seriously damage the offspring if used during pregnancy. Gallbladder disease and adverse effects similar to those of oral contraceptives, including thromboembolism, can occur with estrogenic therapy. (See sections on oral contraceptives.)

LITERATURE

Murad, F, Haynes, RC, Jr. Estrogens and progestins. In The Pharmacological Basis of Therapeutics, 6th ed (Gilman, AG, Goodman, LS, Gilman, A, eds). New York, Macmillan, 1980, Chapter 61.

PROVERA® (Upjohn)
Medroxyprogesterone acetate

1981:169
1980:179
1979:173

Provera is a derivative of progesterone. In women with adequate endogenous estrogen, this compound transforms proliferative into secretory endometrium. Androgenic and anabolic effects have been noted, but the drug appears to be devoid of significant estrogenic activity. While parenterally administered medroxyprogesterone acetate inhibits gonadotropin production, which in turn prevents follicular maturation and ovulation, available data indicate that this action does not occur when the usually recommended oral dose is given as a single daily dose.

INDICATIONS	In secondary amenorrhea, and in dysfunctional uterine bleeding due to hormonal imbalance in the absence of organic pathology.
PREPARATIONS	Tablets: 2.5 and 10 mg.
DOSAGE	Secondary amenorrhea: 5–10 mg daily for 5–10 days. Abnormal bleeding due to hormonal imbalance in the absence of organic pathology: begin on the calculated 16th or 21st day of the menstrual cycle 5–10 mg daily for 5–10 days. See package insert for other indications and dosages.
CONTRAINDICATIONS AND PRECAUTIONS	Provera should not be used in patients with the following conditions: thrombophlebitis, thromboembolic disorders and cerebral apoplexy or a history of these conditions, liver dysfunction or disease, known or suspected breast or genital malignancy, undiagnosed vaginal bleeding, missed abortion, or known sensitivity to medroxyprogesterone. Usage should be discontinued at the earliest manifestations of thrombotic disorders, papilledema retinal vascular lesions and other visual prob-

lems or migraine. Provera is not recommended for use during pregnancy. Provera should be used with caution in nursing mothers.

ADVERSE REACTIONS

In general the adverse effects of progestin therapy resemble those observed with the use of oral contraceptives although the latter are used at higher doses. Breast tenderness or galactorrhea has been reported rarely; sensitivity reactions are occasionally reported. Thromboembolic phenomena have also been reported. Provera therapy may also cause breakthrough bleeding, changes in menstrual flow, amenorrhea, edema, weight changes, cervical secretions and erosions, cholestatic jaundice, rash, and mental depression. For other possibly associated effects see the entries on oral contraceptives and the package insert on Provera.

LITERATURE

Strickler, RC: Postgrad Med 66(5):135, 1979 (dysfunctional uterine bleeding); Wentz, AC: Clin Obstet Gynecol 20:461, 1977 (assessment of estrogen and progestin therapy).

PYRIDIUM® (Parke-Davis)
Phenazopyridine HCl

1981:137
1980:146
1979:144

Pyridium has an analgesic action on the urinary tract and relieves symptoms of dysuria, frequency, burning, and urgency.

INDICATIONS

Pyridium is indicated for the relief of pain, burning, urgency, and frequency, arising from irritations of the lower urinary tract mucosa.

265

PREPARATIONS	Tablets: 100 and 200 mg.
DOSAGE	Average adult dosage is 200 mg three times a day after meals.
CONTRAINDICATIONS AND PRECAUTIONS	Not for use in patients with renal insufficiency.
ADVERSE REACTIONS	Occasional gastrointestinal disturbances, and headache, Methemoglobinemia, hemolytic anemia, and renal and hepatic toxicity have been described, but usually are associated with overdosage. (Urine may turn reddish-orange, but this is not a contraindication.)
LITERATURE	Forland, M: Texas Med 71:70, 1975 (on urinary tract infection management); Green, ED, et al. JACEP 8:426, 1979 (on toxicity and overdose).

QUIBRON® (Mead Johnson)
Theophylline
Guaifenesin

1981:195
1980:173
1979:161

Theophylline, a bronchodilater, acts by direct relaxation of bronchial smooth muscle. It is also a coronary vasodilator, cardiac stimulant, skeletal muscle stimulant, central nervous system stimulant, and diuretic. Guaifenesin increases respiratory tract secretions, possibly by stimulating the Goblet cells.

| INDICATIONS | Quibron is indicated for the symptomatic treatment of bronchospasms associated with such conditions as bronchial asthma, chronic bronchitis, and pulmonary emphysema. It is available in two strengths known as Quibron and Quibron-300, the latter having exactly twice the concentrations of the constituent compounds. |

266

PREPARATIONS	Capsules (soft gelatin); theophylline 150 mg and guaifenesin 90 mg. Liquid: each tablespoon (15 ml) contains theophylline 150 mg and guaifenesin 90 mg. (Quibron-300 has exactly twice the strength of Quibron, but is available only in capsule form). Sustained-release forms are available. (See company literature and Medical Letter reference and Williams, RL et al 1982.)
DOSAGE	Treatment should be *initialized* at 16 mg/kg/day or 400 mg/day whichever is smaller. The usual adjusted doses are adults: 1–2 capsules or 1–2 tablespoons liquid every 6–8 hours. In children the dosage is based on theophylline dose according to weight and age: 9–12 years of age: 4–5 mg theophylline/kg every 6–8 hours; under 9 years of age; 4–6 mg theophylline/kg every 6–8 hours. (See package insert for maximum daily doses in adults and children.)
CONTRAINDICATIONS AND PRECAUTIONS	Quibron is contraindicated in patients with known hypersensitivity to the components or xanthine derivatives. Use cautiously in patients with cardiovascular disease, cor pulmonale, severe hypoxemia, hyperthyroidism, hepatic disease, peptic ulcer, alcoholism, and in the elderly. Concurrent antibiotics (troleandomycin, erythromycin, and clindamycin) and cimetidine may increase serum theophylline levels.
ADVERSE REACTIONS	Gastrointestinal disturbances, CNS stimulation, tachycardia, hypotension, and other cardiovascular effects may occur. Other reported side effects include increased excretion of renal tubular cells and red blood cells, albuminuria, diuresis, tachypnea, hyperglycemia, and inappro-

priate ADH syndrome. Among 245 patients using Quibron and similar theophylline combinations studied in the Boston Collaborative Drug Surveillance Program 18 patients had adverse reactions as follows: gastrointestinal disturbances (13), CNS stimulation (2), tachycardia (1), sensitivity reactions (1), and "other" (1).

LITERATURE

Bergner, RK, Bergner, A. JAMA 235:288, 1976; Hendeles, L, et al: Am J Dis Child 132:876, 1978; Medical Letter 23: 97, 1981; Weinberger, M, Hendeles, L: Postgrad Med 61:85, 1977; Williams, RL, et al. Curr Ther Res 31:45, 1982.

QUINIDINE SULFATE

1981:105
1980:121
1979:126

Quinidine, the dextrostereoisomer of quinine, is a cardiac antiarrhythmic drug. It decreases the firing rate of cardiac Purkinje fibers, increases the diastolic threshold in Purkinje fibers, atrial, and ventricular muscle cells, and also increases the fibrillation threshold in the atria and ventricles. The effective refractory period of these cells is also increased. The conduction velocity in atrial muscle is decreased. Quinidine has a prominent anticholinergic action and alpha-adrenergic blocking actions that can cause vasodilation and hypotension, thereby reflexly activating sympathetic activity that can increase heart rate.

INDICATIONS

Quinidine sulfate is indicated in the treatment of premature atrial and ventricular contractions, paroxysmal supraventricular tachycardia, paroxysmal AV junction rhythm, and paroxysmal ventricular tachycardia when not associated with complete heart block. Quinidine has traditionally been used to convert atrial flutter and fibrillation to sinus rhythm; however, since the advent of DC conversion, quinidine now is used for maintenance therapy in the management of these arrhythmias.

PREPARATIONS

Capsules: 180 and 200 mg. Tablets: 180, 200, and 300 mg. (Extended-release-tablets are usually available—300 mg.)

DOSAGE

The usual adult dosage range is 200–400 mg every 6 hours; the dose in children is 6 mg/kg body weight every 4–6 hours. When quinidine is used in larger daily doses continuous electrocardiographic monitoring is advisable. Elderly patients and those with impaired hepatic or renal function or congestive heart failure may require lower doses. The usual adult dosage for extended release tablets (*adults only*) is 300 or 600 mg every 8 to 12 hours as needed and tolerated.

CONTRAINDICATIONS AND PRECAUTIONS

Contraindications include history of thrombocytopenic purpura associated with quinidine, digitalis intoxication manifested by AV conduction disorders, complete AV block with an AV nodal or idioventricular pacemaker, ectopic impulses, and rhythms due to escape mechanisms or hypersensitivity to the drug. Quinidine should be used very cautiously when there is incomplete AV block, when the patient is digitalized, has congestive failure, or is in a hypotensive state.

ADVERSE REACTIONS

Diarrhea, nausea, and vomiting are the most frequent adverse reactions. Various arrhythmias, hypotension, and other cardiac toxic reactions can occur. Fever, hepatitis, manifestations of cinchonism, blood dyscrasias, and dermatologic reactions occur occasionally. Among 625 patients on quinidine studied in the Boston Collaborative Drug Surveillance Program 89 patients had adverse reactions as follows: gastrointestinal disturbances (44), arrhythmias (21), hypotension (2), other cardiac reactions (4), sensitivity reactions (13), and CNS disturbances (5).

Quinidine interacts with anticoagulants, barbiturates, curariform drugs, digitalis, phenytoin, and rifampin.

LITERATURE

Bigger, JT: Adv Int Med 18:251, 1972; Braunwald, E: In Harrison's Principles of Internal Medicine, 9th ed (Isselbacher, KJ, et al, eds). New York, McGraw-Hill, 1980, Chapter 38; Greenblatt, DJ: J Pharmacol Exp Ther 202:365, 1977; Sodermark, T, et al: Br Heart J 37:486, 1975; White, D, et al. Circulation 56(Suppl 3): 180, 1977.

REGROTON® (USV)
Chlorthalidone
Reserpine

1981:192
1980:170
1979:167

The pharmacologic effects of Regroton are those of the constituent drugs. Chlorthalidone, a potent diuretic, produces a saluretic effect that begins 2 hours after an oral dose and continues for as long as 72 hours. Extensive diuresis is produced with greatly increased excretion of sodium and chloride. Reserpine reduces arterial pressure and exerts a sedative effect. In that sense, it is indicated in the therapy of hypertension with related emotional disturbances.

INDICATIONS

Treatment of hypertension. This combination drug is not indicated for *initial* therapy of hypertension.

PREPARATIONS

Tablets: chlorthalidone 50 mg and reser-

270

pine 0.25 mg. (Demi-Regroton contains half the amount of these components.)

DOSAGE   One Regroton tablet daily (or one Demi-Regroton daily) is the usual adult dosage range.

CONTRAINDICATIONS AND PRECAUTIONS   Mental depression, known hypersensitivity, and most cases of renal or hepatic disease are contraindications. Use cautiously in pregnant women and nursing mothers.

ADVERSE REACTIONS   Gastrointestinal disturbances, nasal congestion, muscle cramps, dizziness, weakness, headache, and mental depression are the most frequent side effects. The side effects of reserpine are well known; however, this preparation contains a much lower concentration of reserpine than that usually implicated in these side effects.

LITERATURE   Finnerty, FA, Jr, et al: JAMA 241:579, 1979; Medical Letter 23:45, 1981; Veterans Administration Cooperative Study Group on Antihypertensive Agents: JAMA 237:2303, 1977.

SALUTENSIN® (Bristol)
Hydroflumethiazide
Reserpine

1981:161
1980:165
1979:172

Salutensin combines two hypertensive agents. Hydroflumethiazide, one of the benzothiadiazides, is an oral diuretic antihypertensive agent. It exerts its effects by inhibiting renal tubular reabsorption, inducing increased excretion of sodium chloride and water with variable losses of potassium and bicarbonate. Reserpine owes its antihypertensive effects to depletion of tissue stores of catecholamines from peripheral site. Reserpine also has a central depleting action that gives it sedative and tranquilizing properties.

INDICATIONS	Salutensin is used in the treatment of hypertension.
PREPARATIONS	Tablets: reserpine 0.125 mg and hydroflumethiazide 50 mg. Demi-tablets: reserpine 0.125 mg and hydroflumethiazide 25 mg.
DOSAGE	The usual adult dosage is 1 regular tablet once or twice daily. When smaller amounts of the diuretic are desired 1 demi-tablet once or twice daily may be given. The precise dosage should be titrated to the needs of the individual patient. Fixed combinations such as Salutensin should not be used as *initial* therapy.
CONTRAINDICATIONS AND PRECAUTIONS	Salutensin should not be used in patients with the following conditions: anuria, oliguria, active peptic ulcer, ulcerative colitis, or severe depression. It is also contraindicated in patients receiving electroconvulsive therapy and in those with hypersensitivity to its components. It is contraindicated in nursing mothers and should be used in women of childbearing age only when the potential benefits outweigh the possible hazards. Salutensin should be used with caution in patients with the following conditions: impaired renal function, hepatic cirrhosis, a history of allergy or bronchial asthma, or systemic lupus erythematosus. Salutensin should be used with caution in patients receiving other antihypertensives concomitantly.
ADVERSE REACTIONS	Adverse reactions of hydroflumethiazide may include hypokalemia, elevation of uric acid, hyperglycemia, and other effects typical of the thiazides. The adverse reactions of reserpine, often transient, include sedation, nightmares, nasal congestion, headache or vertigo, and mental depression. Reserpine interacts with general an-

272

esthetics and with sympathomimetic amines. Thiazides interact with corticosteroids, curariform drugs, digitalis, indomethacin, and lithium.

LITERATURE   Elkowitz, EB: J Am Geriatrics Soc 27:507, 1979; Finnerty, FA: JAMA 241:579, 1979; Medical Letter 23:45, 1981.

SEPTRA® (Burroughs Wellcome)
Trimethoprim
Sulfamethoxasole

1981:122
1980:128
1979:142

The combination of a folic acid antagonist and a sulfonamide inhibits two consecutive steps in the biosynthesis of nucleic acids and proteins essential to many bacteria. The two compounds are synergistic against many common urinary and other type infections.

INDICATIONS   For urinary tract infections, prostatitis, shigellosis, *Pneumocystis carinii* pneumonitis, and typhoid fever resistant to both ampicillin and chloramphenicol. It is also used for treating acute otitis media in children due to susceptible strains of *H. influenzae* or *S. pneumoniae* and acute exacerbations of chronic bronchitis in adults due to these microorganisms.

PREPARATIONS   Tablets sulfamethoxazole 400 mg and trimethoprim 80 mg.
(See SEPTRA DS).

SEPTRA® DS (Burroughs Wellcome)
Trimethoprim
Sulfamethoxasole

1981: 83
1980: 88
1979:116

Septra DS is double strength Septra. The combination of a folic acid antagonist and a sulfonamide inhibits two consecutive steps in the biosynthesis of nucleic acids and proteins essential to many bacteria. The two compounds are synergistic against many common urinary and other type infections.

INDICATIONS

For urinary tract infections, prostatitis, shigellosis. *Pneumocystis carinii* pneumonitis, and typhoid fever resistant to both ampicillin and chloramphenicol. It is also used for treating acute otitis media in children due to susceptible strains of *H. influenzae* of *S. pneumoniae* and acute exacerbations of chronic bronchitis in adults due to these microorganisms.

PREPARATIONS

Tablets: sulfamethoxazole 800 mg and trimethoprim 160 mg. The oral suspension contains sulfamethoxazole 200 mg and trimethoprim 40 mg per 5 ml (teaspoon).

DOSAGE

For adults the usual dosage for urinary tract infections is 1 Septra DS tablet or 2 Septra tablets every 12 hours for 10 to 14 days. The same dosage is used for 5 days in the treatment of shigellosis. The usual dosage for children with urinary tract infections or acute otitis media is 8 mg/kg trimethoprim and 40 mg/kg sulfamethoxazole per day given in two divided doses every 12 hours for 10 days (5 days for treating shigellosis). For patients with renal impairment half the usual dose is used. For cases of severe renal impairment (creatinine clearance below

15 ml/min) this drug is not recommended. For treating acute exacerbations of chronic bronchitis in adults the usual dosage is 1 Septra DS tablet or 2 Septra tablets (or 4 teaspoons) every 12 hours for 14 days. For treating pneumocystis carinii pneumonitis the usual adult dose is based on patient weight: 20 mg/kg trimethoprim and 100 mg/kg sulfamethoxazole per day given in equally divided doses every 6 hours for 14 days. In children weighing 80 lb (36 kg) the dosage is 1 Septra DS tablet every 6 hours for 14 days. For children less than 80 lb consult the package insert or equivalent company literature.

CONTRAINDICATIONS AND PRECAUTIONS

Septra should not be used by pregnant women, nursing mothers, infants less than 2 months of age, or patients with hypersensitivity to trimethoprim or sulfonamides. Septra should not be used in the treatment of streptococcal pharyngitis. Septra should be discontinued if the blood count is significantly reduced.

ADVERSE REACTIONS

Gastrointestinal disturbances, allergic reactions, and blood dyscrasias can occur. Central nervous system reactions including muscle weakness have been reported as have drug fever, chills, and toxic nephrosis with oliguria and anuria. Periarteritis nodosa and lupus-like phenomena have occurred. Sulfonamides can increase the anticoagulant effect of warfarin and can also enhance the action of oral hypoglycemics.

LITERATURE

Finland, M, Kass, EH (eds): J Infect Dis 128(Suppl):425, 1972 (see also Drugs 1:7, 1971); Kunin, CM, et al: JAMA 239:2588, 1978, Lau, WK, Young, LS: N Engl J Med 295:716, 1976; Medical Letter 23:69,

1981, 23:102, 1981; Wormser, GP: NY
State J Med 78:1915 and 2058, 1978.

SER-AP-ES® (Ciba)   1981:71
Hydralazine HCl   1980:73
Reserpine   1979:62
Hydrochlorothiazide

Ser-Ap-Es is a combination of three antihypertensives. Hydralazine
is a direct vascular smooth muscle relaxing agent. Hydrochlorothiazide is a diuretic that also relaxes vascular smooth muscle, and reserpine lowers blood pressure by depleting catecholamine stores.

INDICATIONS	Hypertension: not for initial therapy, but in more severe cases that do not respond satisfactorily to monotherapy.
PREPARATIONS	Tablets: reserpine 0.1 mg, hydralazine hydrochloride 25 mg, and hydrochlorothiazide 15 mg.
DOSAGE	The usual dosage is 1 or 2 tablets three times daily. (Adjustment to the lowest effective dose in the individual patient should be made. Reserpine effects may not become maximal for 2 weeks.)
CONTRAINDICATIONS AND PRECAUTIONS	Ser-Ap-Es should not be used in patients with the following conditions: mental depression, active peptic ulcer, ulcerative colitis, coronary artery disease, mitral valvular rheumatic heart disease, anuria, or hypersensitivity to any of the ingredients. Ser-Ap-Es should be used with caution in patients with the following conditions: renal disease, liver disease, a history of allergy or bronchial asthma, or systemic lupus erythematosus. Ser-Ap-Es should be

used with extreme caution in patients receiving MAO inhibitors or other antihypertensives concomitantly.

ADVERSE REACTIONS

The most common adverse effects of hydralazine are headache, vertigo, gastrointestinal disturbances, tachycardia, and
palpitation. A lupus-like syndrome may
develop with chronic high doses. Reserpine may cause drowsiness, headache,
vertigo, nasal stuffiness, and depression;
other effects are infrequent. The most frequent effects of hydrochlorothiazide are
hypokalemia, hyponatremia, hyperuricemia, and gastrointestinal disturbances.
(See also APRESOLINE and HYDRO-
CHLOROTHIAZIDE.)

LITERATURE

Bello, CT, et al: J Clin Pharmacol 14:630,
1974; David, NA, et al: Curr Ther Res
18:741, 1975; Medical Letter 23:45, 1981.

SERAX® (Wyeth)
Oxazepam

1981:100
1980: 99
1979:100

Oxazepam, from the class of benzodiazepines, is used to control
common emotional disturbances. It exerts rather prompt action in
a wide variety of disorders associated with anxiety, tension, agitation,
irritability, and in anxiety associated with depression. This drug has
a shorter half-life than most other benzodiazepines.

INDICATIONS

Serax is indicated for the management
and control of anxiety disorders or for
the short-term relief of the symptoms of
anxiety. The anxiety associated with depression is responsive to Serax. It is said
to be particularly useful in the manage-

277

ment of anxiety, tension, irritability, and agitation in older patients. Tension associated with alcohol withdrawal is responsive to Serax.

<table>
<tr><td>PREPARATIONS</td><td>Capsules: 10, 15, and 30 mg. Tablets: 15 mg.</td></tr>
<tr><td>DOSAGE</td><td>Adults: 30–120 mg daily in three or four divided doses depending on severity of symptoms; elderly patients: initially 30 mg daily divided into three doses; if necessary, this dosage may be gradually increased to 45–60 mg daily in three or four divided doses. (Information on children under 12 years is inadequate; not for children under 6 years of age.)</td></tr>
<tr><td>CONTRAINDICATIONS AND PRECAUTIONS</td><td>Serax should not be used by pregnant women or patients with psychosis or a history of hypersensitivity to oxazepam. Serax should be used with caution in patients receiving other CNS depressants concomitantly. It should also be used cautiously in patients in whom a drop in blood pressure could lead to cardiac complications.</td></tr>
<tr><td>ADVERSE REACTIONS</td><td>The frequency of untoward effects is low. Drowsiness is the most common. Less frequently seen are rash, nausea, dizziness, syncope, hypotension, tachycardia, edema, nightmares, and other CNS reactions. Blood reactions and liver dysfunction have been rarely reported. Large doses may lead to dependence.</td></tr>
<tr><td>LITERATURE</td><td>Ayd, FJ, Jr (ed). Proc. Conf. Oxazapam. Dis Nerv Sys 36(5):Section 2, 1975; Medical Letter 23:41, 1981 (choice of benzodiozepines).</td></tr>
</table>

SINEQUAN® (Roerig)
Doxepin HCl

1981:79
1980:79
1979:80

Doxepin, from the class of tricyclic antidepressants, inhibits reuptake of biogenic amines in the CNS; however, this action alone does not adequately explain its antidepressant effect.

INDICATIONS

Sinequan is indicated in the treatment of psychoneurotic patients with depression and/or anxiety, in patients with depression and/or anxiety associated with alcoholism (not to be taken with alcohol) and in depression and/or anxiety associated with organic diseases. It is also indicated in psychotic depressive disorders with associated anxiety including involutional depression and manic-depressive disorders. Drugs in this class do not produce mood elevation in normal patients.

PREPARATIONS

Capsules: 10, 25, 50, 75, 100, and 150 mg of doxepin. Solution (concentrate): 10 mg of doxepin per ml.

DOSAGE

The dosage for adult patients with mild to moderately severe illness, is initially 75–150 mg daily in divided doses. This dosage may be increased, for more severely ill patients, gradually to 300 mg daily if necessary. In patients with very mild symptoms, or emotional symptoms accompanying organic disease, doses as low as 25–50 mg/day may suffice. If a once-a-day dosing schedule is used, the maximum dose is 150 mg/day and may be given at bedtime. *The 150 mg capsule strength is intended for maintenance only and not for initiating therapy.*

CONTRAINDICATIONS AND PRECAUTIONS	Sinequan should not be used in patients with the following conditions: glaucoma, tendency to urinary retention, or hypersensitivity to dibenzoxepines. Sinequan should not be used by pregnant women, children under 12, or patients receiving MAO inhibitors concomitantly. Sinequan should be used with extreme caution in patients who may use alcohol excessively.
ADVERSE REACTIONS	Sedation and anticholinergic effects (dry mouth, blurred vision, and constipation) are the most common. Cardiac and CNS effects may occur with higher doses. Allergic reactions, blood dyscrasias, endocrine effects, and jaundice are less common. Interactions with barbiturates, clonidine, guanethidine, levodopa, MAO inhibitors, phenytoin, and sympathomimetic amines occur.
LITERATURE	Ananth, JV, et al: Curr Ther Res 25:133, 1979 (geriatric use); Int Drug Therapy Newsletter 14:1, 1979 (review of 10 years' experience).

SLO-PHYLLIN® GYROCAPS® (Dooner)
Theophylline, anhydrous

1981:173
1980:199
1979: —

Theophylline is a xanthine bronchodilator. Like other xanthines it also has cardiac positive inotropic, vasodilating, and diuretic actions. It is an inhibitor of cyclic nucleotide phosphodiesterase. Slo-phyllin capsules are in timed-release form in a special base that provides for a prolonged therapeutic effect.

INDICATIONS	Slo-phyllin is used in the treatment of asthma and other pulmonary disorders in which a reversible bronchoconstrictive el-

ement may be present such as chronic bronchitis and emphysema.

PREPARATIONS

Timed-release capsules: 60, 125, and 250 mg.

DOSAGE

Initial Dose: 16 mg/kg/day or 400 mg/day (whichever is lower) in 2 or 3 divided doses at 8–12 hour intervals. This dosage may be increased in 25% increments at 2–3 day intervals, if no intolerance is observed, until the following maxima (based on age and ideal body weight) are reached: Age 6 months to 9 years—24 mg/kg/day; Age 12 years to 16 years—18 mg/kg/day; Age > 16 years—13 mg/kg/day or 900 mg/day, *whichever is less.*

CONTRAINDICATIONS AND PRECAUTIONS

Slo-phyllin should not be used in patients who have demonstrated hypersensitivity to xanthines; not for concomitant use with other xanthines. Slo-phyllin should be used with extreme caution in pregnant women and patients with the following conditions: peptic ulcer, lowered body plasma clearance, liver dysfunction, and chronic obstructive lung disease.

ADVERSE REACTIONS

Headache, dizziness, nervousness, vomiting, and epigastric pain are common. CNS stimulation, palpitation, fall in blood pressure, diuresis, with possible increased excretion of red blood cells, renal tubular cells and albumin, tachypnea, hyperglycemia and inappropriate ADH syndrome may occur. Among 256 patients on various theophylline preparations studied in the Boston Collaborative Drug Surveillance Program 25 patients had side effects as follows: gastrointestinal disturbances (15), tachyarrhythmias (4), vertigo (2), sensitivity reactions (2), and "other" (2). Theophylline interacts with furosemide, hexamethonium, reserpine, cimetidine,

281

erythromycin, propranolol, troleandomycin, and influenza vaccine.

LITERATURE   Bell, T, Bigley, J: Pediatrics 62:352, 1978; Medical Letter 23:97, 1981; Weinberger, M, et al: N Engl J Med 299:852, 1978; Wilson, AE, McPhillips, JJ. Annu Rev Pharmacol Toxicol 18:541, 1978.

SLOW-K® (Ciba)
Potassium chloride

1981:23
1980:26
1979:31

Potassium ion is the principal intracellular cation of most body tissues. Its concentration may diminish whenever the rate of potassium loss through renal excretion and also through the gastrointestinal tract exceeds the rate of potassium intake. This depletion may develop as a consequence of prolonged therapy with oral diuretics, primary or secondary hyperaldosteronism, diabetic ketoacidosis, severe diarrhea, or inadequate replacement of potassium in patients on prolonged parenteral nutrition.

INDICATIONS

For therapeutic uses in patients with hypokalemia with or without metabolic alkalosis, in digitalis intoxication, and in patients with hypokalemic familial periodic paralysis. It is also used for the prevention of potassium depletion when the dietary intake of potassium is inadequate in conditions of digitalis and diuretics for congestive heart failure, in hepatic cirrhosis with ascites, and in other states in which potassium depletion occurs. It is probably not needed by the patient receiving diuretics for uncomplicated essential hypertension if the dietary intake of potassium is normal. *Because of reports of intestinal and gastric ulceration with slow-release potassium chloride, these drugs should be reserved for those*

*patients who cannot take liquid or effervescent
potassium preparations.*

PREPARATIONS

Sugar-coated tablets: potassium chloride
600 mg (8 mEq).

DOSAGE

The dosage must be individualized but
is usually in the range of 20 mEq daily
for prevention of hypokalemia to 40–100
mEq daily for treatment of potassium depletion.

CONTRAINDICATIONS
AND PRECAUTIONS

Slow-K should not be used in patients
with the following conditions: hyperkalemia, enlarged left atrium, metabolic acidosis, or any condition delaying gastrointestinal transit. Slow-K should not be used
in conjunction with potassium-sparing diuretics. Potassium salts should be used
with caution by individuals with chronic
renal disease or impaired potassium excretion. Slow-K should be discontinued
immediately if severe vomiting, abdominal pain, distention, or gastrointestinal
bleeding occur.

ADVERSE REACTIONS

The most common side effects are hyperkalemia, nausea, vomiting, abdominal discomfort, and diarrhea. Among 6797 patients receiving potassium chloride
(several forms and routes) in the Boston
Collaborative Drug Surveillance Program
410 patients had adverse reactions as follows: hyperkalemia (259), gastrointestinal
disturbances (109), injection site complications, phlebitis (32), arrhythmias (3),
pain (2), hematemasis (1), and "other"
(4).

LITERATURE

Lubbe, WF, et al; NZ Med J 90(647):377,
1979; Medical Letter 20(6): 30, 1978;
Medical Letter 23:3, 1981; Moleski, R,
Borruso, RD: Hosp Pharm 12:311, 1977;
Page, C: Med News 11(38):10, 1979.

SORBITRATE® (Stuart)
Isosorbide dinitrate

1981:127
1980:133
1979:150

Isosorbide dinitrate, an organic nitrate, relaxes smooth muscle and is used for the relief of angina pectoris and for prophylaxis in situations likely to provoke such attacks. The precise mechanism in the relief of angina pectoris is not known.

INDICATIONS

The sublingual and chewable forms of Sorbitrate are indicated for treatment of the acute anginal attack and for prophylaxis in situations likely to provoke such attacks. The oral dosage form of Sorbitrate is not intended to abort the acute anginal episode but is possibly effective for prophylaxis. (Oral nitrates are under investigation for possible use in treating congestive heart failure. See Franciosa et al, 1978; Hardarson et al, 1977; Aronow, 1980.)

PREPARATIONS

Chewable tablets: 5 and 10 mg. Tablets: 5, 10, and 20 mg. Sustained action tablets: 40 mg. Sublingual tablets: 2.5 and 5 mg.

DOSAGE

The smallest effective dose should be used, especially with chewable forms, since severe hypotensive responses may occur. The individual oral dose is 2.5 to 10 mg, although doses up to 30 mg have been used, and may be taken 3–4 times daily. The sustained action tablet may be taken at 12 hr intervals. Chewable and sublingual forms are used as needed or at 4 to 6 hour intervals.

CONTRAINDICATIONS AND PRECAUTIONS

Sorbitrate should not be used in patients with a history of sensitivity to the drug. Nitrates should be used with extreme caution during the early days of the acute phase of myocardial infarction.

ADVERSE REACTIONS

Headache is the most common untoward reaction. Dizziness, vertigo, weakness, and other signs of postural hypotension are seen less frequently. Gastrointestinal disturbances, restlessness, pallor, perspiration, and collapse occur in some sensitive individuals. Among 361 patients on isosorbide dinitrate studied in the Boston Collaborative Drug Surveillance Program 34 patients had adverse effects as follows: headache (27), vertigo (3), gastrointestinal disturbances (3), and hypotension (1).

LITERATURE

Aronow, WS: J Cardiovasc Med 5:157, 1980; Franciosa, JA, et al: JAMA 240:443, 1978; Hardarson, T, et al: Am J Cardiol 40:90, 1977; Klaus, AP, et al: Circulation 48:519, 1973; Thadani, U, et al: Circulation 61:526, 1980.

STELAZINE® (Smith Kline & French)
Trifluoperazine HCl

1981:151
1980:153
1979:141

Trifluoperazine is a potent tranquilizer from the phenothiazine group. Like other phenothiazines, trifluoperazine has antiemetic action. As a group, the phenothiazines produce emotional quieting, psychomotor slowing, and affective indifference. They tend to decrease paranoid ideation, anxiety, delusions, and agitation. Hypotension and sedation are less likely with Stelazine than with some of the other phenothiazines, but all of these cause Parkinson-like symptoms.

INDICATIONS

For the management of the manifestation of psychotic disorders. It is possibly useful in controlling excessive anxiety, tension, and agitation as seen in neuroses or associated with somatic conditions.

285

PREPARATIONS

Tablets: 1, 2, 5, and 10 mg. Multiple-dose vials: 2 mg/ml. Concentrate (for institutional use only): 10 mg/ml.

DOSAGE

The oral dose for adult outpatients is 2–4 mg daily in divided doses; in hospitalized patients the oral dose for adults is *initially* 4–10 mg daily in divided doses (with gradual increments to the optimal dose). Elderly or debilitated patients should receive ⅓ to ½ of the above doses. The oral dose for children 6 years or older is 1–2 mg daily, gradually increased to an optimal amount (usually not more than 15 mg daily). The intramuscular route can be used for prompt control of severe symptoms. In adults, initially 1–2 mg, followed by 1–2 mg every 4–6 hours, not to exceed 10 mg daily. Elderly and debilitated patients should receive ⅓ to ½ of the above dose. In children 6 years or older the intramuscular dose is 1 mg, once or twice daily (based on limited experience). Oral administration is recommended when symptoms are controlled.

CONTRAINDICATIONS AND PRECAUTIONS

Stelazine should not be used in patients who are comatose or in greatly depressed states due to CNS depressants. Stelazine should not be used by individuals with the following conditions: existing blood dyscrasias, bone marrow depression, preexisting liver damage, or a history of hypersensitivity to phenothiazines. Stelazine should be used with caution in pregnant women and in patients receiving CNS depressants concomitantly. There is evidence that phenothiazines are excreted in the breast milk of nursing mothers.

ADVERSE REACTIONS

Extrapyramidal effects, convulsions, altered CNS fluid proteins, cerebral edema, and autonomic reactions (dry mouth, nasal congestion, headache, gastrointestinal effects, inhibition of ejaculation) can occur. Occasionally blood dyscrasias or jaundice occur. Ocular changes have been noted. (For other adverse reactions see the company literature.) Phenothiazines interact with barbiturates, guanethidine, levodopa, lithium, phenytoin, and propranolol; they may diminish the effect of oral anticoagulants.

LITERATURE

Baldessarini, RJ: In The Pharmacological Basis of Therapeutics, 6th ed (Gilman, AG, Goodman, LS, Gilman, A. eds). New York, Macmillan, 1980, Chapter 19; Bernstein, JG: Drug Ther 9:71, 1979 (prescribing antipsychotics); Blau, S: J Clin Psychiatry 39(10):766, 1978 (guide to psychotropic medication in children and adolescents); Hall, P: Practitioner 219: 493, 1977 (choice of medical treatment of schizophrenia).

STUARTNATAL 1 + 1® TABLETS (Stuart)

1981:193
1980:180
1979: —

Stuartnatal 1 + 1 is a vitamin and mineral supplementation preparation. It contains folic acid to aid in the prevention of megaloblastic anemia.

INDICATIONS

To provide vitamin and mineral supplementation throughout pregnancy and during the postnatal period for both lactating and nonlactating mothers.

PREPARATIONS

The composition of each tablet is as follows: vitamins A (8000 IU), D (400 IU), E (30 IU), and C (90 mg), folic acid (1 mg), thiamine mononitrate (2.55 mg), riboflavin (3 mg), niacinamide (20 mg), B_6 as pyridoxine HCl (10 mg) and B_{12} (12 μg). Minerals: calcium (200 mg), iodine (150 μg), iron (65 mg), magnesium (100 mg).

DOSAGE

One tablet daily after a meal.

CONTRAINDICATIONS AND PRECAUTIONS

None known.

ADVERSE REACTIONS

None known (Note: FD&C Yellow #5 has been eliminated from this product.)

LITERATURE

The Pharmacological Basis of Therapeutics, 6th ed (Gilman, AG, Goodman, LS, Gilman, A, eds). New York, Macmillan, 1980, pp 1551–1601.

SULAMYD® Sodium (Schering)
Sulfacetamide sodium ophthalmic

1981:189
1980:193
1979: —

Sulamyd is a bacteriostatic agent effective against a wide range of gram-positive and gram-negative microorganisms.

INDICATIONS

Sulamyd sodium is indicated for the treatment of conjunctivitis, corneal ulcer, and other superficial ocular infections. It is also an adjunct to systemic sulfonamide therapy of trachoma.

PREPARATIONS

Solutions (aqueous): 10 and 30% sulfacetamide sodium and sodium thiosulfate 1.5 mg/ml plus preservatives (methylparaben 0.5 mg/ml and propylparaben 0.1 mg/ml) and sodium dihydrogen phosphate buffer. Ointment (10%): in each gram sulfacetamide sodium 100 mg plus preservatives (methylparaben 0.5 mg,

<table>
<tr><td></td><td>propylparaben 0.1 mg, and benzalkonium chloride 0.25 mg) and sorbitan monolaurate and water.</td></tr>
<tr><td>DOSAGE</td><td>Ophthalmic solution 10%: 1 or 2 drops into the lower conjunctival sac every 2 or 3 hours during the day and less often at night. Ophthalmic ointment 10%: a small amount is applied four times daily and at bedtime. Ophthalmic solution 30%: for conjunctivitis or corneal ulcer, 1 drop into lower conjunctival sac every 2 hours (less frequently in milder cases); for trachoma, 2 drops every 2 hours; concomitant systemic sulfonamide therapy is indicated.</td></tr>
<tr><td>CONTRAINDICATIONS AND PRECAUTIONS</td><td>Known hypersensitivity to sulfonamides or to any ingredient in these preparations is a contraindication. These preparations are incompatible with silver preparations. Nonsusceptible organisms may proliferate with the use of these agents.</td></tr>
<tr><td>ADVERSE REACTIONS</td><td>Local irritation may occur. Burning and stinging has been reported with the 30% solution; sensitivity reactions may occur but are rare.</td></tr>
<tr><td>LITERATURE</td><td>Gottschalk, HR, Stone, OJ: Arch Dermatol 112:513, 1976; Medical Letter 22:96, 1980.</td></tr>
</table>

SUMYCIN® (Squibb)
Tetracycline HCl

1981:135
1980:117
1979: 92

Tetracyclines are mainly bacteriostatic and are thought to exert their antimicrobial effect by the inhibition of protein synthesis in a wide range of gram-negative and gram-positive organisms. Tetracyclines are readily absorbed and bind to plasma proteins.

INDICATIONS

Tetracyclines are indicated in infections caused by the following: Rickettsiae, *Mycoplasma pneumonia,* agents of psittacosis and ornithosis, agents of lymphogranuloma venereum and granuloma inguinale, and the spirochetal agent of relapsing fever (*Borrelia recurrentis*). The following gram-negative micro-organisms are also sensitive: *Haemophilus ducreyi, Pasteurella* species, *Bartonella bacilliformis, Bacteroides* species, *Vibrio comma* and *Vibrio fetus* and *Brucella* species (in conjunction with streptomycin). *Tetracyclines* are alternates to penicillin in treating infections due to: *Neisseria gonorrhea, Treponema pallidum* and *Treponema pertenue, Listeria, Clostridium, Bacillus anthracis, Fusobacterium fusiforme* (Vincent's infection) and *Actinormyces* species. Certain other gram-positive and gram-negative microorganisms may be treated with tetracyclines when bacteriologic testing indicates appropriate susceptibility. *Tetracyclines* are usually not useful in streptococcal diseases; they have been successfully used in the management of acne. Other indications are in the treatment of trachoma and in inclusion conjunctivitis.

PREPARATIONS

Tablets or capsules: 250 and 500 mg. Syrup: in each 5 ml (teaspoon), 125 mg tetracycline hydrochloride buffered with potassium metaphosphate.

DOSAGE

Oral. Adults: usual daily dose is 1–2 g. Children over 8 years: 25–50 mg/kg body weight daily in four divided doses. Therapy should continue for 24–48 hours after signs and symptoms disappear. Streptococcal infections should be treated for at least 10 days.

For treatment of gonorrhea, 1–5 g initially, then 0.5 g every 6 hours until a total of 9 g have been given. For treatment

290

of syphilis, a total of 30–40 g, in equally divided doses over a period of 10–15 days is used. When used for severe acne, 1 g daily in divided doses, for 1 week, then reduced gradually to maintenance levels of 125–500 mg daily.

CONTRAINDICATIONS AND PRECAUTIONS

Known hypersensitivity to any tetracycline is a contraindication. Caution must be exercised in patients with renal or hepatic problems. The use of tetracyclines during the last half of pregnancy (tooth development phase) may lead to permanent discoloration of the teeth of the offspring. Infants and children under 8 years who use these drugs can experience tooth discoloration.

ADVERSE REACTIONS

Gastrointestinal disturbances (nausea and vomiting) are the most common adverse effects; tooth discolorations (as described above) can occur. Less frequent adverse reactions include malabsorption, enterocolitis, photosensitivity and various sensitivity reactions. Superinfection, rise in BUN and renal damage may occur. Other reactions occur, but are rare. Among 1172 patients on tetracyclines studied in the Boston Collaborative Drug Surveillance Program 73 patients had adverse reactions as follows: gastrointestinal disturbances (41), superinfection (9), rise in BUN (8), sensitivity reactions (8), injection site complications (5), and "other" (2). These drugs interact with oral antacids, bismuth subsalicylate, oral contraceptives, oral iron, methoxyflurane and zinc sulfate. Because tetracyclines may depress plasma prothrombin activity, patients on anticoagulant therapy may require lower doses of the anticoagulant.

LITERATURE

Am Acad Dermatol (Ad Hoc Committee

291

on Antibiotics): Arch Dermatol 111:1630, 1975; Finland, M: Clin Pharmacol Ther 15:3, 1974 (commentary of tetracyclines); Johnson, AH: Semin Drug Treat 2:331, 1972 (adverse effects); Medical Letter 24:21, 1982 (choice of antimicrobials). Siegel, D: NY State J Med 78:950 and 1115, 1978 (reviews on tetracyclines).

SYNALAR® (Syntex)
Fluocinolone Acetonide

1981:185
1980:184
1979:179

Synalar is a topical steroid primarily effective because of its anti-inflammatory, antipruritic, and vasoconstrictive actions.

INDICATIONS	For the relief of inflammatory manifestations of corticosteroid-responsive dermatoses.
PREPARATIONS	Creams: 0.025% and 0.01%. Ointment: 0.025%. Topical solution: 0.01%. Also available as a cream: 0.2% called Synalar-HP.
DOSAGE	A sparing amount is applied to the affected area three to four times daily and gently rubbed in. With occlusive dressings, application is directly to the affected area, leaving a thin surface coating. Changes of dressing may be made one or two times a day.
CONTRAINDICATIONS AND PRECAUTIONS	Topical steroids are contraindicated in those patients with a history of hypersensitivity to any of the components of the preparation (see product insert for list of components). Treatment should be discontinued if irritation develops. Safety in

292

pregnant women has not been established. Use with caution in the presence of infection, and when treating children and infants, especially when used with an occlusive dressing (since systemic absorption may occur). Topical steroids are not for ophthalmic use. Synalar-HP should not be used in infants up to 2 years.

ADVERSE REACTIONS   Irritation may develop.

LITERATURE   Stoughton, RB: In Recent Advances in Dermatopharmacology (Frost, P, et al. eds). New York, Spectrum, 1978, pp 105–112.

SYNALGOS-DC® (Ives)   1981:91
Dihydrocodeine bitartrate   1980:86
Promethazine HCl   1979:97
Aspirin
Caffeine

Dihydrocodeine is a semisynthetic narcotic analgesic related to codeine with multiple actions qualitatively similar to those of codeine. The most prominent of these involve the central nervous system and organs with smooth muscle components. The principal actions of therapeutic value are analgesia and sedation. Promethazine is a phenothiazine with sedative actions. Synalgos also contains the nonnarcotic antipyretic analgesic combination aspirin-caffeine.

INDICATIONS   Possibly effective for the relief of moderate to moderately severe pain in those situations in which a mild sedative effect is desired.

PREPARATIONS   Capsules: dihydrocodeine bitartrate 16.0 mg, promethazine HCl 6.25 mg, aspirin 356.4 mg, and caffeine 30.0 mg.

293

DOSAGE	Usual adult dosage is 2 capsules every 4 hours as needed for pain.
CONTRAINDICATIONS AND PRECAUTIONS	Hypersensitivity to dihydrocodeine, promethazine or aspirin is a contraindication. Aspirin should be used with caution in the presence of peptic ulcer or coagulation abnormalities. Psychic dependence, physical dependence, and tolerance may develop upon repeated administration of dihydrocodeine. Use with care in the presence of other CNS depressants. Safety for use during pregnancy, nursing, or in children has not been established.
ADVERSE REACTIONS	Most frequently seen are drowsiness, dizziness, sedation, nausea, vomiting, constipation, pruritis, and skin reactions. Hypotension may occur, but is rare. Dihydrocodeine may be habit forming.
LITERATURE	AMA Drug Evaluations, 4th ed. New York, AMA and Wiley, 1980, pp 84–85.

SYNTHROID® (Flint)
Levothyroxine sodium

1981:30
1980:34
1979:37

Synthroid, available as tablets and injections, contains a synthetic levothyroxine, the principal hormone secreted by the normal thyroid gland. Taken orally, Synthroid provides hormone that is readily absorbed from the gastrointestinal tract. The injection is effective by any parenteral route.

INDICATIONS	Synthroid is a specific replacement therapeutic agent used for reduced or absent thyroid function of any etiology.
PREPARATIONS	Tablets: 25, 50, 100, 150, 200 and 300 μg. Injection: 10 ml vials containing 100

294

mcg, 200 mcg and 500 mcg of lyophilized active ingredient, 10 mg of mannitol, USP and 0.7 mg tribasic sodium phosphate anhydrous (must be reconstituted by adding 5 ml of 0.9% sodium chloride injection, USP or bacteriostatic sodium chloride injection, USP with benzyl alcohol only).

DOSAGE

For treating mild hypothyroidism, in young and middle-aged adults, the initial dose is 50–100 μg daily, with increments of 50–100 μg at 2–3 weeks intervals if necessary until the desired response is obtained. For most adults a final dosage of 100–200 μg is sufficient, and 400 μg daily is a practical upper limit. (Failure to respond to 400 μg is rare and should prompt reconsideration of the diagnosis.) The recommended daily replacement dosage in children is: 0–1 year: 9 mcg/kg; 1–5 years: 6 mcg/kg; 6–10 years: 4 mcg/kg; 11–20 years: 3 mcg/kg. Dose is administered once daily only. (See Fisher, 1978.) In myxedema coma or stupor, 200–500 μg may be given I.V., followed on the next day by 100–300 μg. Not to be added to other IV fluids. (See package insert for further information.)

CONTRAINDICATIONS AND PRECAUTIONS

Acute myocardial infarction, uncorrected adrenal insufficiency, and thyrotoxicosis are contraindications. Large doses, used in the treatment of obesity, may cause serious side effects, particularly when given in the presence of sympathomimetic amines (see product insert for details). The 100 and 300 μg tablets contain FD&C Yellow #5 which may cause allergic-type reactions (frequently seen in patients who are allergic to aspirin).

ADVERSE REACTIONS

The untoward effects follow from overdose and are those that resemble hyper-

thyroidism. Thyroid hormones interact
with oral anticoagulants, cholestyramine,
and tobramycin.

LITERATURE

DeGroot, LJ, Niepomniszcze, H: Metabolism 26:665, 1977; Fisher, DA: Thyroid Today 1(8):1, 1978; Jackson, IMD, Cobb, WE: Am J Med 64:284, 1978.

TAGAMET® (Smith Kline & French)
Cimetidine

1981: 9
1980:15
1979:22

Tagamet is a histamine H_2 receptor antagonist that is used in the
treatment of ulcers and other conditions characterized by excesses
of gastric acid secretions. This drug inhibits the action of histamine
at the histamine (H_2) receptors of the parietal cells and also inhibits
gastric acid secretion stimulated by food, histamine, caffeine, insulin,
and pentagastrin. Tagamet is not an anticholinergic drug. The use
of H_2 receptor antagonists represents a new method of treatment
of peptic ulcer and Tagamet is the first drug in this class.

INDICATIONS

Tagamet is indicated in the short-term
treatment of active duodenal ulcer (up to
8 weeks) and for prophylactic use in
duodenal ulcer patients (at reduced dosage) to prevent ulcer recurrence in patients who, based on history of recurrence
or complications, are likely to need surgery. It is also indicated in the treatment
of pathologic hypersecretory conditions.

PREPARATIONS

Tablets: 200 and 300 mg. Injectable
forms: vials of concentration 300 mg/2
ml. Liquid: 300 mg/5ml.

DOSAGE

The recommended adult oral dosage for
duodenal ulcer is 300 mg four times a
day, with meals and at bedtime. Treatment should normallly be continued for

4–6 weeks. For treating hypersecretory conditions, the recommended adult oral dosage is 300 mg four times a day, with meals and at bedtime, and should be continued as long as clinically indicated (not to exceed 2400 mg daily).

When the oral form cannot be used or is undesirable parenteral routes are used. For intravenous use 300 mg is diluted with sodium chloride injection (0.9%) to a volume of 20 ml and injected over a period not less than 2 minutes and is administered every 6 hours. Intermittent intravenous infusions may be used (see package insert). For intramuscular injection: 300 mg (without dilution) every six hours. Experience in children is limited; hence the benefits and risks should be carefully considered before instituting therapy with Tagamet in children. For patients with severely impaired renal function the recommended dosage (based on limited experience) is 300 mg every 12 hours, orally or intravenously, with adjustment (cautiously).

CONTRAINDICATIONS

There are no known contraindications to the use of Tagamet; however, usage in pregnant and nursing women is limited and, thus, caution should be taken in these patients.

ADVERSE REACTIONS

Among 9907 patients treated with Tagamet the reported incidences of side effects were as follows: gastrointestinal (2.1%), central nervous system (dizziness, headache, and sleepiness, 1.2%), and skin allergies (0.5%). Most of these were mild and transient. Less frequently observed adverse effects were as follows: gynecomastia, musculoskeletal, urinary tract, dry mouth, taste and vision disturbances, chest pain and palpitation, and blood reactions. Cimetidine has been reported to increase blood levels of phenytoin, propranolol, chlordiazepoxide, diazepam and thephylline, and to increase bone marrow depression with carmustine.

LITERATURE

Brogden, RN, et al: Drugs 15:93, 1978 (review of cimetidine in peptic ulcer disease); Burland, WL, Simkins, MA, eds: Proc Second Int Symposium on Histamine H_2-Receptor Antagonists: Cimetidine. Amsterdam, Exerpta Medica, 1977; Cheli, R, et al: Curr Ther Res 30:1039, 1981 (continuous treatment at low dosage); Hirschowitz, BI: Annu Rev Pharmacol Toxicol 19:203, 1979 (H_2 receptors). Romankiewicz, JA, Reidenberg, MM: Rational Drug Ther 15(5), May, 1981 (review).

TALWIN® (Winthrop)
Pentazocine HCl

1981:114
1980: 95
1979: 88

Pentazocine, from the benzomorphan group, is a potent analgesic. When administered orally (50 mg) its analgesic effect is approximately the same as 60 mg of codeine. Pentazocine is a weak antagonist of morphine, meperidine, and phenazocine. It also has sedative activity.

INDICATIONS

Talwin is used for relief of moderate to severe pain.

PREPARATIONS

Tablets: equivalent to 50 mg pentazocine. (Also available as injection and as Talwin compound which contains 325 mg aspirin.)

DOSAGE

Usual adult dosage range of Talwin tablets is 1–2 every three to four hours when needed, not to exceed 600 mg daily. Usage in children under 12 years of age is not recommended. (For parenteral uses see package insert.)

CONTRAINDICATIONS
AND PRECAUTIONS

Talwin is contraindicated in patients known to be sensitive to pentazocine hydrochloride. Psychic dependence, physical dependence, and tolerance have been reported upon repeated administration of parenteral pentazocine in patients with a history of drug abuse. Use with caution in patients with obstructive respiratory conditions, or impaired renal or hepatic function. Safety for use during pregnancy, nursing, or in children has not been established.

ADVERSE REACTIONS

The untoward effects after oral pentazocine include neuropsychiatric and other CNS effects, gastrointestinal disturbances, sweating and other autonomic effects, and allergic reactions. Less frequently seen are tachycardia, decrease in blood pressure, hematologic reactions, respiratory depression, urinary retention, paresthesia, and toxic epidermal necrolysis. Dependence and withdrawal symptoms may occur. Among 616 patients receiving oral pentazocine studied by the Boston Collaborative Drug Surveillance Program 17 patients had adverse reactions as follows: gastrointestinal disturbances (constipation) (4), neuropsychiatric effects including hallucinations (4), disorientation (1), bizarre feelings (1), vertigo (3), nightmares (1), dry mouth (2), and sensitivity reactions (1).

LITERATURE

Brogden, RN, et al: Drugs 5:6, 1973; Lewis, JR, JAMA 225:1530, 1973.

TENUATE® (Merrell-National)
Diethylpropion HCl

1981:115
1980: 98
1979: 87

Tenuate, used to treat obesity, is a sympathomimetic amine with some pharmacologic activity similar to the amphetamines. Its actions include some central nervous system stimulation and elevation of blood pressure. Tolerance has been demonstrated with all drugs of this class.

INDICATIONS	Tenuate is indicated in the management of exogenous obesity as a short-term adjunct in a regimen that includes weight reduction based on caloric restriction.
PREPARATIONS	Tablets: 25 mg. Timed-release tablets: 75 mg.
DOSAGE	The usual adult oral dose is 25 mg three times daily 1 hour before meals; an additional 25 mg may be taken in the evening if needed. An alternate schedule is 1 timed-release tablet (75 mg) taken in mid-morning.
CONTRAINDICATIONS AND PRECAUTIONS	Tenuate is contraindicated in patients with the following conditions: advanced arteriosclerosis, hyperthyroidism, known hypersensitivity, or idiosyncrasy to the sympathomimetic amines, and glaucoma. It is also contraindicated in patients in agitated states, patients with a history of drug abuse, and during or within 14 days following the administration of MAO inhibitors (hypertensive crises may result). Psychic dependence may develop to this amphetamine-like drug. If tolerance develops the drug should be discontinued. Safety for use during pregnancy has not been established and use in children under 12 years of age is not recommended.

ADVERSE REACTIONS Mild restlessness, dry mouth, and constipation are common. Other side effects include nervousness, excitability, euphoria, and insomnia. Psychic dependence may occur.

LITERATURE Craddock, D: Drugs 11:378, 1976. Jasinski, DR, et al: Clin Pharmacol Ther 16:645, 1974; McQuarrie, HG: Curr Ther Res 17:437, 1975; Nolan, GR: Curr Ther Res 18:332, 1975.

TETRACYCLINE SYSTEMIC

1981:10
1980: 8
1979: 7

Tetracyclines are mainly bacteriostatic and are thought to exert their antimicrobial effect by the inhibition of protein synthesis in a wide range of gram-negative and gram-positive organisms. Tetracyclines are readily absorbed and bind to plasma proteins.

INDICATIONS Tetracyclines are indicated in infections caused by the following: Rickettsiae, *Mycoplasma pneumonia*, agents of psittacosis and ornithosis, agents of lymphogranuloma venereum and granuloma inguinale, and the spirochetal agent of relapsing fever (*Borrelia recurrentis*). The following gram-negative micro-organisms are also sensitive: *Haemophilus ducreyi*, *Pasteurella* species, *Bartonella bacilliformis*, *Bacteroides* species, *Vibrio comma* and *Vibrio fetus* and *Brucella* species (in conjunction with streptomycin). *Tetracyclines* are alternates to penicillin in treating infections due to: *Neisseria gonorrhea*, *Treponema pallidum* and *Treponema pertenue*, Listeria, Clostridium, Bacillus anthracis, Fusobacterium fusiforme (Vin-

301

cent's infection) and *Actinomyces* species. Certain other gram-positive and gram-negative microorganisms may be treated with tetracyclines when bacteriologic testing indicates appropriate susceptibility. *Tetracyclines* are usually not useful in streptococcal diseases; they have been successfully used in the management of acne. Other indications are in the treatment of trachoma and in inclusion conjunctivitis.

PREPARATIONS

Capsules: 250 and 500 mg. Syrup: 125 mg/5 ml. Powder: 250 and 500 mg for IV use. (See also ACHROMYCIN V, SUMYCIN, MINOCIN, VIBRAMYCIN.)

DOSAGE

Oral. Adults: usual daily dose is 1–2 g. Children over 8 years: 25–50 mg/kg body weight daily in four divided doses. *Intravenous.* Adults: 250–500 mg twice daily at 12 hour intervals. Children over 8 years: 20–30 mg/kg body weight daily in divided doses every 8–12 hours. The intramuscular route can be very painful and is generally not used. Therapy should continue for 24–48 hours after signs and symptoms disappear. Streptococcal infections should be treated for at least 10 days.

For treatment of gonorrhea, 1.5 g (orally) initially, then 0.5 g every 6 hours until a total of 9 g have been given. For treatment of syphilis, a total of 30–40 g (orally), in equally divided doses over a period of 10–15 days is used. When used for severe acne, 1 g (orally) daily in divided doses for 1 week, then reduced gradually to maintenance levels of 125–500 mg daily.

CONTRAINDICATIONS
AND PRECAUTIONS

Known hypersensitivity to any tetracycline is a contraindication. Caution must be exercised in patients with renal or hepatic

302

problems. The use of tetracyclines during the last half of pregnancy (tooth development phase) may lead to permanent discoloration of the teeth of the offspring. Infants and children under 8 years who use these drugs can experience tooth discoloration.

ADVERSE REACTIONS

Gastrointestinal disturbances (nausea and vomiting) are the most common adverse effects; tooth discoloration (as described above) can occur. Less frequent adverse reactions include malabsorption, enterocolitis, photosensitivity, and various sensitivity reactions. Superinfection, rise in BUN, and renal damage may occur. Other reactions occur, but are rare. Among 1172 patients on tetracyclines studied in the Boston Collaborative Drug Surveillance Program 73 patients had adverse reactions as follows: gastrointestinal disturbances (41), superinfection (9), rise in BUN (8), sensitivity reactions (8), injection site complications (5), and "other" (2). These drugs interact with oral antacids, bismuth subsalicylate, oral contraceptives, oral iron, methoxyflurane, and zinc sulfate. Because tetracyclines may depress plasma prothrombin activity, patients on anticoagulant therapy may require lower doses of the anticoagulant.

LITERATURE

Am Acad Dermatol (Ad Hoc Committee on Antibiotics): Arch Dermatol 111:1630, 1975; Finland, M: Clin Pharmacol Ther 15:3, 1974 (commentary on tetracyclines); Johnson, AH: Semin Drug Treat 2:331, 1972 (adverse effects); Medical Letter, 24:21, 1982 (choice of antimicrobials); Siegel, D: NY State J Med 78:950 and 1115, 1978 (reviews on tetracyclines).

THEO-DUR® (Key)
Theophylline (sustained-release)

1981: 76
1980:118
1979: —

Theophylline is a xanthine bronchodilator. Like other xanthines it also has cardiac positive inotropic, vasodilating, and diuretic actions. It is an inhibitor of cyclic nucleotide phosphodiesterase. Theo-dur tablets are in timed-release form and should not be chewed or crushed.

INDICATIONS	Theo-dur is used for symptomatic relief and/or prevention in patients with asthma and other pulmonary disorders such as bronchitis and emphysema in which reversible bronchospasm is present.
PREPARATIONS	Sustained-release tablets: 100, 200, and 300 mg.
DOSAGE	Children weighing 15–20 kg: one 100 mg tablet every 12 hours; children weighing 20–25 kg: one-half (150 mg) of a 300 mg tablet every 12 hours; children weighing 25 kg or more: one 200 mg tablet every 12 hours. The average initial adult dosage is one 300 mg tablet every 12 hours. Dosage levels should be individualized because of variable rates of elimination among patients.
CONTRAINDICATIONS AND PRECAUTIONS	Patients with known hypersensitivity to xanthines should not use this preparation; not for use concomitantly with other xanthines. This drug should be used cautiously in pregnant women and in patients with the following conditions: peptic ulcer, lowered body plasma clearance, liver dysfunction, and chronic obstructive lung disease.
ADVERSE REACTIONS	Headache, dizziness, nervousness, vomiting, and epigastric pain are common. CNS

304

stimulation, palpitation, fall in blood pressure, and diuresis may occur. Among 256 patients on various theophylline preparations studied in the Boston Collaborative Drug Surveillance Program 25 patients had side effects as follows: gastrointestinal disturbances (15), tachyarrhythmias (4), vertigo (2), sensitivity reactions (2), and "other" (2). Theophylline interacts with furosemide, hexamethonium, reserpine, cimetidine, erythromycin, propranolol, troleandomycin, and influenza vaccine.

LITERATURE   Bell, T, Bigley, J: Pediatrics 62:352, 1978; Medical Letter 23:97, 1981; Weinberger, M. et al: N Engl J Med 299:852, 1978; Wilson, AE, McPhillips, JJ: Annu Rev Pharmacol Toxicol 18:541, 1978.

THORAZINE® (Smith Kline & French)   1981:108
Chlorpromazine HCl   1980:101
                                         1979: 86

Chlorpromazine, a potent tranquilizer, is the prototype of the phenothiazine group of psychotropic agents. Although the principal pharmacologic actions are psychotropic, it also has sedative and antiemetic activity. Chlorpromazine acts at all levels of the central nervous system. It has strong antiadrenergic and weaker peripheral anticholinergic activity.

INDICATIONS   Thorazine is used for the management of manifestations of psychotic disorders and in the control of nausea and vomiting. It is also used to control manifestations of manic-depressive illness and to treat intractable hiccups. Prior to surgery, thorazine is useful to control restlessness and apprehension. It is used for control of intermittent porphyria and as an adjunct in the treatment of tetanus. Thorazine is useful to control moderate or severe agitation and hyperactivity and aggressiveness in disturbed children.

PREPARATIONS

Tablets: 10, 25, 50, 100, and 200 mg. Capsules (sustained release "Spansules"): 30, 75, 150, 200, and 300 mg. Ampuls: 1 and 2 ml containing 25 mg/ml. Multiple-dose vials: 10 ml vials containing 25 mg/ml. Syrup: each 5 ml (teaspoon) contains 10 mg. Suppositories: 25 and 100 mg. Concentrate: 30 and 100 mg/ml.

DOSAGE

Psychiatric Use Oral: For adult outpatients, 30–75 mg daily in 2 or 3 divided doses. For severe psychosis in adults the initial dose is 25 mg 3 times a day. This dose is increased if necessary after 1–2 days until symptoms are controlled. In elderly or debilitated patients one-third to one-half the usual dose is used and increases should be more gradual. For children the dose is 0.5 mg/kg body weight every 4–6 hours. In severe cases in hospitalized children daily doses of 50–200 mg may be necessary. *Intramuscular:* for acutely psychotic hospitalized adults, 25–100 mg initially, repeated in 1–4 hours if necessary. Most patients respond to a daily dose of 0.5–1 g although daily dosage of up to 1.6 g, in divided doses, might be needed for control. Oral dosages are used when the patient becomes calm. In children, 0.5 mg/kg body weight every 6–8 hours with gradual increments if necessary (not to exceed 40 mg daily in children under 5, or 75 mg daily in older children). Oral administration should be used when the symptoms are controlled. The *intravenous* route is irritating and should not be used. The rectal route is used in children:

1mg/kg body weight every 6–8 hours. (For dosage information in other conditions, consult package insert.)

CONTRAINDICATIONS AND PRECAUTIONS

Thorazine is contraindicated in individuals in comatose states, in the presence of large amounts of CNS depressants (alcohol, barbiturates, narcotics, etc.), and in the presence of bone marrow depression. Thorazine should be avoided in patients with signs and symptoms that suggest Reye's syndrome, or with known hypersensitivity to phenothiazines. Safety during pregnancy or nursing has not been established.

ADVERSE REACTIONS

Sedation, dry mouth, blurred vision, urinary retention, and constipation are common. In older patients especially the incidence of dizziness, hypotension, ophthalmic changes, and dyskinesias is high. Mild photosensitivity occurs relatively often. Agranulocytosis and cholestatic jaundice occur rarely. Phenothiazines interact with barbiturates, guanethidine, levodopa, lithium, phenytoin, and propranolol. Among 556 patients on chlorpromazine studied in the Boston Collaborative Drug Surveillance Program 68 patients had adverse effects as follows: drowsiness, ataxia, or confusion (32), hypotension (12), respiratory depression (4), possible hepatotoxicity (4), sensitivity reactions (3), estrapyramidal reactions (3), coma (2), tachycardia (2), cardiac arrest (1), hematologic toxicity (1), seizure (1), and "other" (3).

LITERATURE

Baldessarini, R: In The Pharmacological Basis of Therapeutics 6th ed (Gilman, AG, Goodman, LS, Gilman, A eds). New York, Macmillan, 1980, Chapter 19 (pharmacology and therapeutic uses of phenothi-

307

azines); Clark, ML, et al: Psychopharm Bull 14:43, 1976 (kinetics and clinical response); Dahl, SG, Strandjord, RE: Clin Pharmacol Ther 21:437, 1977 (pharmacokinetics); Hernandez, LL, Appel, JB: Psychopharmacology 60:125, 1979 (perceptual effects); Linden, R, et al: N Engl J Med 296:1004, 1977 (tardive dyskinesia); Swazey, JP: Minn Med 62:81, 1979 (historical) Weintraub, M, Barry, DJ: Drug Ther 9:99, 1979 (management of agitated aggressive patient).

THYROID

1981:47
1980:58
1979:54

Thyroid hormones have their major effects on metabolism, growth and development. These effects are exerted through the control of protein synthesis. They are calorigenic, that is, the rate of cellular oxidation is increased, thereby increasing energy utilization and heat production. Their protein anabolic effect is important in normal growth and development. Thyroid is prepared from cleaned, defatted, dessicated thyroid glands of edible animals.

INDICATIONS

Thyroid is used in the treatment of thyroid deficiency states, especially cretinism and myxedema. Thyroid is also indicated as adjunctive therapy when thyroid-inhibiting agents are used.

PREPARATIONS

Capsules: 60, 120, 180, 240, and 300 mg. Tablets: 15, 30, 60, 90, 120, 240, and 300 mg. Chewable tablets: 180 mg. Tablets (enteric and timed-release): 30, 120, and 200 mg.

DOSAGE

For replacement therapy in *young adults* the dosage range is usually 15–30 mg daily initially, with increments of 15–20 mg at

2 week intervals until the desired response is obtained. For maintenance, 60–120 mg daily in a single dose is used. For *older adults*, initially 7.5–30 mg daily; this dose is doubled at 6–8 week intervals until the desired response is obtained. For suppressive therapy the initial dose is lower and gradually increased as required to a daily maintenance dose of 90–180 mg.

CONTRAINDICATIONS AND PRECAUTIONS

Thyroid preparations are contraindicated in the presence of uncorrected adrenal insufficiency and in acute myocardial infarction which is uncomplicated by hypothyroidism. Patients with myxedema may be especially sensitive to thyroid hormones and, therefore, should receive very small doses with gradual (monthly) increments. Thyroid should be used cautiously in patients with cardiovascular disease or diabetes mellitus (insulin or hypoglycemic dosage may require adjustment).

ADVERSE REACTIONS

Excessive doses of thyroid produce signs and symptoms of thyrotoxicosis: tachycardia, arrhythmias, palpitation, elevated pulse pressure, angina pectoris, tremors, nervousness, headache, insomnia, diarrhea, changes in appetite, excessive sweating, and intolerance to heat and fever. Chronic overdosage causes emaciation.

LITERATURE

DeGroot, LJ, Niepomniszcze, H: Metabolism 26:665, 1977; Jackson, IMD, Cobb, WE: Am J Med 64:284, 1978.

TIGAN® (Beecham)
Trimethobenzamide HCl

1981:167
1980:159
1979:159

Tigan is an antiemetic agent. The mechanism of its action is not precisely known but is thought to be related to its effects on the chemoreceptor trigger zone, an area of the medulla through which emetic impulses are conveyed to the vomiting center.

INDICATIONS	For the control of nausea and vomiting.
PREPARATIONS	Capsules: 100 and 250 mg. Suppositories: 200 mg. Pediatric suppositories: 100 mg. Injectable ampuls: 2 ml containing 200 mg. Vials: 20 ml containing 100 mg/ml. Disposable syringes: 2 ml containing 100 mg/ml.
DOSAGE	The usual adult oral dosage is 250 mg three or four times a day. The dosage in children (30–90 lb) is 100–200 mg three or four times daily. The suppositories (200 mg) are used as follows: Adults: 1 suppository (200 mg) three or four times a day. Children: ½ suppository (100 mg) three or four times daily. The pediatric suppositories (100 mg) are useful in children under 30 lb: 1 suppository (100 mg) three or four times a day. Injectable forms are used in adults only: 200 mg three or four times a day via the intramuscular route (preferably the upper outer quadrant of the gluteal region).
CONTRAINDICATIONS AND PRECAUTIONS	The injectable form of Tigan in children, the suppositories in premature or newborn infants, and use in patients with known hypersensitivity to trimethobenzamide are contraindicated. Tigan suppositories contain benzocaine and should not be used in patients known to be sensi-

tive to this or similar local anesthetics. Tigan is not recommended for uncomplicated vomiting in children (see product insert for details). Use with caution in acute febrile illness, encephalitides, gastroenteritis, dehydration, and electrolyte imbalance, especially in children and the elderly. Safety for use during pregnancy or nursing has not been established.

ADVERSE REACTIONS

Gastrointestinal disturbances, sensitivity reactions, and drowsiness may occur but are of low frequency. There have been reports of blood dyscrasias, blurred vision, CNS effects, headaches, jaundice, muscle cramp, and opisthotonos. Among 890 patients on trimethobenzamide studied in the Boston Collaborative Drug Surveillance Program 9 patients had adverse effects as follows: gastrointestinal disturbances (4), sensitivity reactions (2), drowsiness (2), and urinary retention (1).

LITERATURE

Kaan, SK, Eshelman, FN: Curr Ther Res 26:210, 1979.

TIMOPTIC® (Merck Sharp & Dohme)
Timolol maleate

1981:60
1980:64
1979:73

Timolol, an ophthalmic preparation, is a nonselective beta-adrenergic antagonist with little or no agonist activity and no local anesthetic properties. Timoptic ophthalmic solution, when applied topically in the eye, reduces both elevated and normal intraocular pressure. (Timolol was recently released in an oral formulation for treatment of hypertension as well as for use after myocardial infarction. See Medical Letter reference for further information.)

311

INDICATIONS	Timoptic is effective for the reduction of elevated intraocular pressure. It is useful in patients with chronic open-angle glaucoma, patients with aphakic glaucoma, and in certain patients with secondary glaucoma. It is also used in patients with ocular hypertension.
PREPARATIONS	Sterile ophthalmic solution: 5 and 10 ml ophthalmic dispensers with a controlled drop tip, concentrations 0.25% and 0.5%.
DOSAGE	The usual starting dose is 1 drop of 0.25% solution in each eye twice a day. If necessary the dosage may be increased by using 1 drop of the 0.5% solution in each eye twice daily. (See package insert for further details.)
CONTRAINDICATIONS AND PRECAUTIONS	Timoptic is contraindicated in patients who are known to be hypersensitive to any of the components of this product. Because of possible systemic absorption, Timoptic should not be used in patients with known contraindications to systemic use of beta-adrenergic blocking agents (see product insert for details). Safety for use during pregnancy, nursing, or in children has not been established.
ADVERSE REACTIONS	Ocular irritation occurs occasionally. Hypersensitivity reactions (rash and/or urticaria) and visual disturbances may occur, but are rare.
LITERATURE	Boger, WP, III, et al: Am J Ophthalmol 86:8, 1978; Medical Letter 20(25): 109, 1978; Medical Letter 24:43, 1982 (Timolol for use after myocardial infarction and for hypertension); Sonntag, JR, et al: Invest Ophthalmol Visual Sci 17:293, 1978.

TOFRANIL® (Geigy)
Imipramine HCl

1981:150
1980:140
1979:140

Imipramine is the prototype tricyclic antidepressant. The mechanism of its action is not precisely known; it is believed, however, that its antidepressant action is related to enhancement of adrenergic synaptic activity by blocking uptake of norepinephrine at nerve endings.

INDICATIONS	For the relief of symptoms of depression. Endogenous depression is more likely to be alleviated than other depressive states. One to three weeks of treatment may be needed before optimal therapeutic effects are evident. Tofranil may be useful as temporary adjunctive therapy in reducing enuresis in children aged 6 or older, after possible organic causes have been excluded.
PREPARATIONS	Tablets: 10, 25, and 50 mg. Ampuls: 25 mg in 2 ml (1.25%) for intramuscular use only.
DOSAGE	Depression: the usual daily dose in hospitalized patients is initially 100 mg/day in divided doses with a gradual increase, if required, to 200 mg/day. If satisfactory response is not achieved after 2 weeks, the daily dose may be increased to 250–300 mg. For outpatients the initial dose is 75 mg/day with a gradual increase to 150 mg/day. For maintenance of outpatients, 50–150 mg/day. Adolescents and geriatric patients initially receive 30–40 mg/day with increments if necessary (not to exceed 100 mg/day). When the parenteral (I.M.) route is used the initial dose is 100 mg/day in divided doses. (See package insert for uses in children age 6 or

313

older.) Childhood enuresis: initially an oral dose of 25 mg/day one hour before bedtime. If a satisfactory response is not seen within one week, the dose may be increased to 50 mg nightly in children under 12 years; children over 12 years may receive up to 75 mg nightly. Dosage should be reduced gradually when the medication is discontinued.

CONTRAINDICATIONS AND PRECAUTIONS

Use of Tofranil during or within 14 days after administration of MAO inhibitors is contraindicated (hypertensive crises may result). Tofranil is also contraindicated during the acute recovery period after myocardial infarction and in patients with a known hypersensitivity to Tofranil or other dibenzazepines. Extreme caution should be used when given to patients with cardiovascular disease, increased intraocular pressure, hyperthyroidism, and seizure disorders. Tofranil may block the action of guanethidine, clonidine, and similar agents. This drug may enhance the depressant effects of alcohol and other CNS depressants. Safety for use during pregnancy or nursing, has not been established.

ADVERSE REACTIONS

The adverse effects of imipramine commonly include sedation and anticholinergic effects. Cardiac and CNS symptoms may occur in high dosage. Neurological reactions (such as numbness, tingling, and extrapyramidal effects) may occur. Allergic reactions, jaundice, hematologic effects, and endocrine effects occur less often. Abrupt cessation of this drug may produce withdrawal symptoms. Imipramine interacts with barbiturates, clonidine, guanethidine, levodopa, MAO inhibitors, phenytoin, and sympathomimetic amines.

314

LITERATURE

Hollister, LE: N Engl J Med 299:1106, 1978 (tricyclic antidepressants); Orsulak, PJ, Schildkraut, JJ: Ther Drug Monit 1(2): 199, 1979 (monitoring plasma levels); Rosenbaum, AH, et al: Mayo Clin Proc 54(5):335, 1979 (tricyclic agents and MAO inhibitors); Stern, SL, Mendels, J: J Clin Psychiatry 41(2):66, 1980 (withdrawal symptoms).

TOLECTIN® DS (McNeil)
Tolmetin sodium

1981:187
1980: —
1979: —

Tolectin is an anti-inflammatory agent. It has analgesic and antipyretic activity. Although the mechanism of its anti-inflammatory action is not known, Tolectin inhibits prostaglandin synthetase in vitro and lowers the plasma level of prostaglandin E in humans.

INDICATIONS

Tolectin is indicated for the relief of signs and symptoms of rheumatoid arthritis and osteoarthritis. Tolectin is indicated in the treatment of acute flares and the long-term management of the chronic disease. It is also indicated for the treatment of juvenile arthritis.

PREPARATIONS

Tolectin DS capsules: 400 mg. (Also available as Tolectin tablets: 200 mg.)

DOSAGE

Adults: 400 mg three times daily is the recommended starting dose. For rheumatoid arthritis control is usually achieved at doses of 600–1800 mg daily in divided doses; for osteoarthritis, 600–1600 mg daily. Children (2 years or older): 20 mg/kg body weight in three or four divided doses. The usual range after control has been achieved is 15–30 mg/kg daily.

315

Tolectin should not be used in patients who have shown hypersensitivity to tolmetin sodium or to aspirin or other nonsteroidal anti-inflammatory drugs. Use with caution in patients with upper gastrointestinal tract disease, with impaired renal function, and with compromised cardiac function (see package insert for details). Safety for use during pregnancy or nursing has not been established.

ADVERSE REACTIONS

Gastrointestinal symptoms are the most common adverse reactions and range from 1 in 9 patients for nausea to 1 in 55 patients for gastritis. Peptic ulcer occurred in 1 in 50 patients during a large clinical trial with 3000 patients. Other adverse reactions include headache (1 in 10 patients), less frequently, asthenia and chest pain, edema (1 in 15 patients; hypertension less frequently), dizziness and lightheadedness (1 in 20 patients), nervousness (1 in 50 patients), drowsiness (1 in 60 patients; insomnia and depression less frequently), skin rash (1 in 40 patients), pruritis (1 in 60 patients), skin irritation (1 in 55 patients), and tinnitus (1 in 65 patients). A small number of cases of granulocytopenia and anaphylactoid reactions have been reported; decreases in hemoglobin and hematocrit have occurred but these are small and transient.

LITERATURE

Brogden RN, et al: Drugs 15:429, 1978 (review of tolmetin); Symposium: Tolmetin (Ward, JR, ed). Excerpta Medica, 1976.

TOLINASE® (Upjohn)
Tolazamide

1981: 96
1980:111
1979:138

Tolinase is an oral hypoglycemic agent of the sulfonylurea group. These compounds stimulate the islet tissue to secrete insulin. They are ineffective in completely pancreatectomized patients and in insulin-dependent diabetic subjects.

INDICATIONS	The primary indication for tolinase is the stable or maturity-onset type of mild or moderately severe diabetes mellitus.
PREPARATIONS	Tablets: tolazamide 100, 250, and 500 mg.
DOSAGE	For the newly diagnosed adult-onset diabetic, diagnosed as mild to moderately severe, the starting range is 100–250 mg given once a day at breakfast. The malnourished or elderly patient is started on 100 mg daily. Close medical supervision is necessary, especially during the first 6 weeks of therapy. When adjustment upward above 500 mg daily is necessary the drug should be given in two daily doses. For information on transferring patients from other oral hypoglycemics or insulin see package insert.
CONTRAINDICATIONS AND PRECAUTIONS	Tolinase is contraindicated in diabetic patients who have infections, severe trauma, uremia, ketosis, acidosis, coma, or who are undergoing surgery. It is also not indicated in juvenile or labile diabetes or in patients with liver, renal or endocrine disease. Safety has not been established during pregnancy.
ADVERSE REACTIONS	During clinical studies with 1784 patients receiving this drug, 2.1% were taken off

317

for adverse reactions. The side effects are the same as those noted with other sulfonylureas; the incidence is low and the reactions are reversed when the drug is discontinued. These include gastrointestinal disturbances, skin reactions, and (rarely) hematopoietic effects. Hypoglycemia, liver toxicity, and miscellaneous CNS effects (dizziness, vertigo, headache) may occur but are infrequent.

LITERATURE

AMA Drug Evaluations, 4th ed. New York, AMA and Wiley, 1980, pp. 750–755; LeBovitz, HE: Diabetes Care 1:189, 1978 (sulfonylurea drugs); Loiudice, TA, Lang, JA: Am J Gastroenterol 69:81, 1978 (hepatic injury).

TRANXENE® (Abbott)
Chlorazepate dipotassium

1981:37
1980:41
1979:44

Tranxene, one of the benzodiazepine group of antianxiety drugs, has the characteristic actions of this group. It has a depressant effect on the central nervous system.

INDICATIONS

Tranxene is indicated for the symptomatic relief of anxiety and tension associated with anxiety disorders. It is also indicated as adjunctive therapy in the management of partial seizures and in the symptomatic relief of acute alcohol withdrawal.

PREPARATIONS

Tablets and capsules: 3.75, 7.5, and 15 mg. Tranxene-SD tablets: 11.25 and 22.5 mg.

DOSAGE

The usual adult dose for the relief of anxiety is 30 mg daily in divided doses (the range is 15–60 mg daily). It may also be given as a single dose at bedtime. The recommended initial dose is 15 mg. In elderly or debilitated patients the initial dosage should be low, 7.5–15 mg daily. For treating the symptoms of acute alcohol withdrawal doses of 60–90 mg daily are used on day 1, 45–90 mg daily on day 2, 22.5–45 mg daily on day 3, and 15–30 mg daily on day 4. These are administered in divided doses. After day 4 the daily dose is gradually reduced to 7.5–15 mg and discontinued when the patient's condition is stable. As an adjunct to antiepileptic drugs the dosage in adults is initially 7.5 mg three times a day, with increase of not more than 7.5 mg every week, not to exceed 90 mg/day. For children 9–12 years: 7.5 mg two times a day with increase, if necessary, of no more than 7.5 mg every week and not to exceed 60 mg/day.

CONTRAINDICATIONS AND PRECAUTIONS

Tranxene is contraindicated in individuals with a known hypersensitivity to the drug and in those with acute narrow-angle glaucoma. Tranxene is not recommended in patients with depressive neuroses or psychotic symptoms. This drug may enhance the depressant effects of alcohol and other CNS depressants. Psychic and physical dependence similar to those noted with barbiturates and alcohol is possible. Safety for use during pregnancy, nursing, or in children has not been established.

ADVERSE REACTIONS

Drowsiness is the most common adverse effect. Less frequently reported (in descending order) are dizziness, gastrointestinal disturbances, nervousness, blurred vision, dry mouth, headache, and mental confusion. Other reported reactions in-

319

clude insomnia, rash, fatigue, ataxia, genitourinary complaints, diplopia, irritability, depression, and slurred speech. Decrease in blood pressure has been observed and there have been reports of abnormal liver and kidney function tests and of a decrease in hematocrit.

LITERATURE   Berchou, RC et al: Neurology 31:1483, 1981 (anticonvulsant action); Charalampous, KD et al: J Clin Pharmacol 13:114, 1973; Fabre, LF, et al: J Int Med Res 7:147, 1979; General Practitioner Research Group. The Practitioner 215:98, 1975; Lapierre, YD: Int J Clin Pharmacol 11:315, 1975; Medical Letter 23:41, 1981 (choice of benzodiazepines); Mielke, DH, et al: Curr Ther Res 19:506, 1976 (acute alcohol withdrawal).

TRIAVIL® (Merck Sharp & Dohme)
Perphenazine
Amitriptyline HCl

1981:74
1980:71
1979:61

Triavil is a broad-spectrum psychotherapeutic agent for the management of outpatients and hospitalized patients with psychoses or neuroses characterized by mixtures of anxiety or agitation with symptoms of depression. Perphenazine is a potent tranquilizer and potent antiemetic. Amitriptyline is an antidepressant with an anxiety-reducing, sedative component to its action.

INDICATIONS   Triavil is used for the treatment of patients with moderate to severe anxiety and/or agitation and depressed moods, for patient with depression in whom anxiety and/or agitation are severe, and in patients with depression and anxiety in association with chronic physical disease.

320

PREPARATIONS	Tablets: Triavil 2–25 contains perphenazine 2 mg and amitryptyline 25 mg. Triavil 4–25, 4–50, 2–10, and 4–10, containing the respective amounts (in mg), of perphenazine and amitryptyline are also available.
DOSAGE	In psychoneurotic patients when anxiety and depression are of such a degree as to warrant combined therapy, 1 tablet of Triavil 2–25 or 4–25 is given three to four times a day for *initial* dosage. In more severely ill patients with schizophrenia, 2 tablets of Triavil 4–25 are given three times a day. After a satisfactory response is obtained (days to weeks), the maintenance dose range is 1 tablet of Triavil 2–25 or 4–25 two to four times daily, or 1 tablet of Triavil 4–50 twice a day.
CONTRAINDICATIONS AND PRECAUTIONS	Use of Triavil during or within 14 days after administration of MAO inhibitors is contraindicated (hypertensive crises may result). Triavil is also contraindicated during the acute recovery period after myocardial infarction, in patients with a known hypersensitivity to phenothiazines or amitriptyline, in the presence of bone marrow depression, and in CNS depression from drugs (barbiturates, alcohol, narcotics, analgesics, antihistamines). Triavil may block the antihypertensive effect of guanethidine and similarly acting compounds. This drug should be used with caution in patients with a history of urinary retention, glaucoma, convulsive disorders, cardiovascular disorders, and hyperthyroidism. Safety for use during pregnancy, nursing, or in children has not been established.
ADVERSE REACTIONS	The adverse reactions reported are those that occur with perphenazine and with

amitriptyline. Perphenazine, a phenothiazine, may produce adverse reactions that are associated with this class: extrapyramidal effects, tardive dyskinesia, skin disorders and other allergic reactions, autonomic reactions, and others. Amitriptyline can cause dizziness, drowsiness, CNS excitation including hallucinations and involuntary movements, anticholinergic effects, headache, tinnitus, cardiac arrhythmias and hypotension. Amitriptyline and perphenazine may interact with other drugs (see Medical Letter reference).

LITERATURE

Collins, AD, Dundas, J: Br J Psychiat 113:1425, 1967; Diamond, S: Psychosomatics 7:371, 1966; Medical Letter 23:17, 1981.

TRI-VI-FLOR® DROPS (Mead Johnson)
Vitamins A, D, C
Fluoride

1981:171
1980:177
1979:164

Tri-Vi-Flor is a vitamin and fluoride supplement which was developed to provide fluoride for children in areas where the fluoride content of drinking water is too low. This preparation may be useful for children whose diets are lacking in vitamins A, D, and C.

INDICATIONS

For prevention of caries in children ages 2–3 years in areas where drinking water contains less than 0.3 ppm fluoride, and for children over 3 years in areas where the drinking water contains 0.3–0.7 ppm fluoride.

PREPARATIONS

Each 1 ml of Tri-Vi-Flor drops supplies vitamins A (1500 IU), D (400 IU), and

C (35 mg), and fluoride (0.5 mg). Tri-Vi-Flor 0.25 mg is also available and contains 0.25 mg of fluoride.

DOSAGE

The usual dose is 1.0 ml daily for children 2 years of age and older.

CONTRAINDICATIONS
AND PRECAUTIONS

Precaution: The physician should monitor fluoride intake of patient to guard against dental fluorosis (see package insert for details).

ADVERSE REACTIONS

Allergic rash and other idiosyncrasies have been rarely reported.

LITERATURE

Hennon, DK, et al: J Am Dent Assoc 95:965, 1977.

TUSSIONEX® (Pennwalt)

Hydrocodone resin complex
Phenyltoloxamine resin complex

1981:198
1980:185
1979: —

Tussionex is an antitussive agent that acts for approximately 12 hours. It contains the narcotic cough suppressant hydrocodone. The phenyltoloxamine resin complex enhances the effect of hydrocodone.

INDICATIONS

Tussionex is used to treat cough.

PREPARATIONS

Capsules, tablets, and in suspension: each capsule, tablet, or 5 ml (teaspoon) of suspension contains 5 mg of hydrocodone and 10 mg of phenyltoloxamine as cationic resin complexes.

DOSAGE

Adults: 1 teaspoon (5 ml), 1 capsule, or 1 tablet every 8–12 hours. Children under 1 year: $\frac{1}{4}$ teaspoon every 12 hours; from 1–5 years: $\frac{1}{2}$ teaspoon every 12 hours; over 5 years: 1 teaspoon every 12 hours.

CONTRAINDICATIONS
AND PRECAUTIONS

Use with caution in young children, especially those with respiratory conditions. Estimation of dosage relative to the age and weight of the child is of great importance. Hydrocodone may be habit-forming.

ADVERSE REACTIONS

Constipation, nausea, facial pruritis, and drowsiness. These occur infrequently and are usually mild.

LITERATURE

Chan, YT, Hays, EE: Am J Med Sci 234:207, 1957; Irwin RS, et al: Arch Int Med 137:1186, 1977 (comprehensive review on cough); Townsend, EH, Jr: N Engl J Med 258:63, 1958.

TUSS—ORNADE® (Smith Kline & French)

Caramiphen edisylate
Phenylpropanolamine HCl

1981:110
1980: 94
1979: 94

Caramiphen is an antitussive; phenylpropanolamine is an antihistaminic.

INDICATIONS

For the relief of coughing and nasal congestion associated with the common cold.

PREPARATIONS

Tuss-Ornade is available in capsules and a liquid. Each capsule contains caramiphen edisylate 40 mg, and phenylpropanolamine HCl 75 mg. Each 5 ml (teaspoon) of liquid contains caramiphen edisylate 6.7 mg, phenylpropanolamine HCl 12.5 mg, and alcohol 5%.

DOSAGE

Spansules (for adults and children over 12 years only): one spansule every 12 hours. Liquid: adults and children over 12 years of age—2 teaspoons every 4 hours (not to exceed 12 teaspoons in 24 hours). Children 6 to 12 years of age—1 teaspoon every 4 hours (not to exceed 6 teaspoons in 24 hours). Children 2 to 6 years—$\frac{1}{2}$ teaspoon every 4 hours (not to exceed 3 teaspoons in 24 hours).

CONTRAINDICATIONS AND PRECAUTIONS

Tuss-Ornade is contraindicated in patients with hypersensitivity to any of its components, severe hypertension, bronchial asthma, and coronary artery disease. Use of this drug during administration of MAO inhibitors is contraindicated. Do not use liquid in children under 15 lb or in children less than six months of age. Do not use capsules in children under 12 years of age. This drug may enhance the depressant effects of alcohol and other CNS depressants. Use with caution in individuals sensitive to FD&C Yellow #5 (frequently seen in patients who also have aspirin sensitivity), and patients with cardiovascular disease, glaucoma, prostatic hypertrophy, and hyperthyroidism. Safety for use during pregnancy and nursing has not been established.

ADVERSE REACTIONS

Drowsiness, dryness of nose, throat, or mouth, nervousness, and insomnia can occur. Other reactions include gastrointestinal disturbances, dizziness, weakness, tightness of chest, anginal pain, irritability, palpitations, headache, tremor, incoordination, difficulty in urination, blood dyscrasias, convulsions, hypertension, hypotension, anorexia, and visual disturbances.

LITERATURE

Irwin, RS, et al: Arch Int Med 137:1186, 1977 (comprehensive review on cough);

Medical Letter 5:11, 1963. Salem, H, Aviado, DM: Am J Med Sci 247:585, 1964.

TYLENOL®/CODEINE (McNeil)
Acetaminophen
Codeine phosphate

1981:4
1980:3
1979:4

Acetaminophen is a non-narcotic analgesic and antipyretic. Codeine is a narcotic with analgesic and antitussive action.

INDICATIONS

Tylenol with codeine, available in four strengths known as Nos. 1, 2, 3, and 4, is useful for the relief of pain. No. 1, 2, or 3 is indicated for the relief of mild to moderate pain, while two No. 3s or one No. 4 is indicated for the relief of moderate to severe pain. Tylenol with codeine elixir is indicated for the relief of mild to moderate pain.

PREPARATIONS

Tablets and elixir: four strengths are available with regard to codeine phosphate content: No. 1 (7.5 mg), No. 2 (15 mg), No. 3 (30 mg), and No. 4 (60 mg). All four strengths contain 300 mg of acetaminophen. Capsules: two strengths of codeine are available; No. 3 contains 30 mg and No. 4 contains 60 mg; both contain 300 mg of acetaminophen. Elixir: each 5 ml (teaspoon) of the elixir contains 12 mg of codeine phosphate and 120 mg of acetaminophen.

DOSAGE

The usual adult dosage is (for Nos. 1, 2, and 3 tablets) 1 or 2 every 4 hours as needed. The No. 4 preparation is used once every 4 hours as needed. The elixir

326

is used orally. For children 3–6 years: 1 teaspoon three or four times daily; 7–12 years: 2 teaspoons three or four times daily. The adult dose of elixir is 1 tablespoon every 4 hours as needed.

CONTRAINDICATIONS AND PRECAUTIONS

This drug is contraindicated in individuals who are hypersensitive to acetaminophen or codeine. Psychic dependence, physical dependence, and tolerance may develop upon repeated administration of codeine. This drug may enhance the depressant effects of alcohol and other CNS depressants. Safety for use during pregnancy, nursing, or in children under the age of 3 has not been established. Do not give tablets to children under the age of 12. (See product insert for precautions.) Codeine may impair the mental or physical abilities required for the performance of potentially hazardous tasks. Caution should be used when prescribing this drug for elderly or debilitated patients, those with severe renal or hepatic dysfunction, hypothyroidism, Addison's disease, prostatic hypertrophy or urethral stricture. The drug may obscure the diagnosis of acute abdominal conditions.

ADVERSE REACTIONS

The most frequent adverse reactions are lightheadedness, dizziness, sedation, shortness of breath, nausea, and vomiting. Other untoward effects include euphoria, dysphoria, constipation, skin rash, and pruritis. The CNS depressant action of this drug may be additive with that of other central depressants. The acetaminophen component has a very low incidence of adverse effects. Among 1215 patients on acetaminophen in the Boston Collaborative Drug Surveillance Program 4 patients had adverse reactions as follows: diaphoresis (2), gastrointestinal disturbance (1), and sensitivity reaction (1). Among 817 patients on oral codeine 29 had adverse effects as follows: constipation (14), nausea or vomiting (7), rash (3), and CNS effects (5).

LITERATURE

Ameer, B, Greenblatt, DJ: Ann Intern Med 87:202, 1977 (acetaminophen); Medical Letter 20:61, 1978 (acetaminophen); Moertel, GC, et al: N Engl J Med 286:813, 1972 (comparative evaluation of codeine and other analgesics).

VALISONE® (Schering)
Betamethasone valerate

1981:87
1980:77
1979:76

Betamethasone, a corticosteroid, has anti-inflammatory, antipruritic, and vasoconstrictive actions. Valisone is available as ointment, lotion, cream, and aerosol.

INDICATIONS

Valisone cream, ointment, and lotion are indicated for the relief of inflammatory manifestations of corticosteroid responsive dermatoses. The aerosol is indicated only for adjunctive topical management of acute contact dermatitis.

PREPARATIONS

Aerosol: 0.15%. Cream: 0.1%. Lotion: 0.1%. Ointment: 0.1%. Reduced strength cream: 0.01%.

DOSAGE

The cream or ointment is applied as a thin film to the affected skin area one to three times a day. The lotion is applied to the affected skin area and massaged lightly until it disappears, twice daily. The aerosol is directed to the affected area at a distance of 6 inches and applied for 3 seconds, three to four times daily.

CONTRAINDICATIONS AND PRECAUTIONS

Topical steroids are contraindicated in those patients with a history of hypersensitivity to any of the components of the preparation (see product insert for list of components). Treatment should be discontinued if irritation develops. Safety in pregnant women has not been established. Use with caution in the presence of infection and when treating children and infants, especially when used with an occlusive dressing (since systemic absorption may occur). Topical steroids are not for ophthalmic use.

ADVERSE REACTIONS

The following have been reported: burning, itching, irritation, dryness, folliculitis, hypertrichosis, acneform eruptions, hypopigmentation, perioral dermatitis, allergic contact dermatitis, maceration of the skin, secondary infection, skin atrophy, striae, and miliaria.

LITERATURE

Stoughton, RB: In Recent Advances in Dermatopharmacology (Frost, P, et al, eds). New York, Spectrum, 1978, pp 105–112.

VALIUM® (Roche)
Diazepam

1981:1
1980:1
1979:1

Diazepam is a member of the benzodiazepine class of antianxiety drugs and may be considered the prototype of its class. Based on animal studies, diazepam appears to act on parts of the brain limbic system, the thalamus, and the hypothalamus. In addition to its tranquilizing effects it has hypnotic, anticonvulsant, and muscle relaxing properties.

329

INDICATIONS

Valium is indicated for the management of anxiety; it is also useful as adjunctive therapy in the relief of skeletal muscle spasm, in acute alcohol withdrawal, and as adjunctive therapy in convulsive disorders.

PREPARATIONS

Tablets: 2, 5, and 10 mg for oral administrations. Ampuls: 2 ml of concentration 5 mg/ml.

DOSAGE

2–10 mg, two to four times daily for relief of tension and anxiety states; in acute alcohol withdrawal, 10 mg, three or four times during first 24 hours, with reduction to 5 mg, three or four times daily as needed subsequently. Lower doses are recommended in geriatric patients and in children. Not for use in children less than 6 months of age. For muscle spasm, 5–10 mg I.M. or I.V. initially and repeat in 3 to 4 hours if necessary. In status epilepticus, 5 to 10 mg I.V. (slowly) initially and repeat in 10–15 minute intervals if necessary up to total 30 mg.

CONTRAINDICATIONS
AND PRECAUTIONS

Valium should not be used in the treatment of psychotic patients, in patients with known hypersensitivity, or in patients with acute narrow angle glaucoma. Not for children under 6 months of age. Valium should be used cautiously in depressed patients, those with impaired renal or hepatic function and patients engaging in tasks that require complete mental alertness.

ADVERSE REACTIONS

Drowsiness is the most common adverse reaction; disorientation and confusion, ataxia, and vertigo can occur; depression, sensitivity reactions, hypotension, and gastrointestinal disturbances can occur, but are rare; other CNS manifestations have been reported, but are of very low frequency. Withdrawal symptoms have been seen following abrupt discontinuance in patients who had received excessive doses over an extended period of time. Interactions with other drugs are rare, although heavy cigarette smoking may reduce its effectiveness. The action of Valium may be potentiated by alcohol, narcotics, barbiturates, MAO inhibitors, and other antidepressants. Cimetidine may reduce the clearance of Valium and other benzodiazepines.

Among 2623 patients on diazepam studied in the Boston Collaborative Drug Surveillance Program 208 patients experienced adverse reactions as follows: drowsiness (119), disorientation (20), ataxia, vertigo or dysarthria (15), depression (9), sensitivity reactions (9), hypotension (9), gastrointestinal disturbances (9), headache (4), respiratory depression (4), coma (3), CNS excitation (4) and "other" (3).

LITERATURE

Medical Letter 15:1, 1973; Medical Letter 23:41, 1981 (choice of benzodiazepines); Rickels et al: Antianxiety drugs: Clinical use in psychiatry. In Handbook of Psychopharmacology 13 (Iverson et al, eds). New York, Plenum Press, 1978, pp 395–430; Garattini, S, et al (eds): The Benzodiazepines, New York, Raven Press, 1973. Sepinwall J, Cook, L. In Handbook of Psychopharmacology 13 (Iverson et al, eds). New York, Plenum Press, 1978, pp 345–393.

VANCERIL® (Schering)
Beclomethasone dipropionate inhaler

1981:179
1980:188
1979: —

Beclomethasone dipropionate, the chlorinated esterified analogue of betamethasone, is a corticosteroid that acts locally on the respiratory mucosa. It is used for patients with asthma who require steroids, and is prepared for *oral* inhalation.

INDICATIONS	This preparation is for use *only* in patients who require chronic treatment with corticosteroids for control of the symptoms of bronchial asthma and should *not* be used for asthma that can be controlled by bronchodilators and other nonsteroidal medications.
PREPARATIONS	Vanceril is available for oral inhalation only in a metered-dose aerosol unit. Each actuation delivers a quantity of 42 μg of beclomethasone dipropionate. The contents of one canister will provide 200 oral inhalations.
DOSAGE	Adults: usually 2 inhalations three or four times a day, not to exceed 20 inhalations per day. Children 6–12 years: usually receive 1 or 2 inhalations three or four times per day, not to exceed 10 inhalations per day.
CONTRAINDICATIONS AND PRECAUTIONS	Vanceril is contraindicated in patients with a known hypersensitivity to any of the components of this preparation, and in the primary treatment of status asthmaticus or other acute episodes of asthma where intensive measures are required. Use extreme caution when transferring patients from systemic corticosteroids to Vanceril (see Warning in product insert). Use with caution in the presence of respi-

ratory infection. Safety for use during pregnancy or nursing has not been established.

ADVERSE REACTIONS

Adrenal insufficiency can occur during and after transfer from systemic corticosteroids to aerosol beclomethasone dipropionate. *Caution should be exercised during the transfer,* with gradual decrements in the dosage of systemic steroid medication. Careful monitoring is necessary. (Consult the package insert for details.) Localized infections with *Candida albicans* or *Aspergillus niger* have occurred frequently in the mouth and pharynx and occasionally in the larynx. A few instances of hoarseness and dry mouth have been reported. Bronchospasm and rash have been reported rarely. The long-term effects of beclomethasone dipropionate in humans are still unknown.

LITERATURE

Ballin, JC: JAMA 236:2891, 1976.

VASODILAN® (Mead Johnson Pharm.)
Isoxsuprine HCl

1981:175
1980:156
1979:149

Isoxsuprine directly dilates vascular smooth muscle. This relaxation may increase blood flow to certain regions.

INDICATIONS

Possibly effective for the relief of symptoms associated with cerebral vascular insufficiency, in peripheral vascular disease of arteriosclerosis obliterans, and in Raynaud's disease. The efficacy of direct vasodilators in the treatment of vascular insufficiency is questionable.

333

PREPARATIONS	Tablets: 10 and 20 mg. Ampuls: 10 mg in 2 ml.
DOSAGE	Oral: 10–20 mg three or four times daily. Intramuscular: 5–10 mg (1–2 ml) two or three times daily.
CONTRAINDICATIONS AND PRECAUTIONS	There are no known contraindications to oral use when administered in recommended doses. Do not give postpartum or in the presence of arterial bleeding. Do not give intravenously. Parenteral administration is not recommended in the presence of hypotension or tachycardia.
ADVERSE REACTIONS	Hypotension, tachycardia, nausea and vomiting, dizziness, abdominal distress, and rash may occur but are rare with oral use. The intramuscular route, in higher doses, may produce hypotension and tachycardia.
LITERATURE	AMA Drug Evaluations, 4th ed. New York, AMA and Wiley, 1980, pp 541–542; Coffman, JD, Mannick, JA: Ann Int Med 76:35, 1972; Strandness, E: JAMA: 213:86, 1970.

V-CILLIN K® (Lilly)
Penicillin V potassium

1981:28
1980:23
1979:20

Penicillin V, the phenoxymethyl analogue of penicillin G, is a semi-synthetic penicillin for *oral* use; discussed here is the potassium salt of penicillin V (often called Penicillin VK). This drug is more stable in acid than is penicillin G and, thus, it is better absorbed from the gastrointestinal tract. Its actions are the same as those of penicillin G for gram-positive microorganisms and it is, therefore, preferable to penicillin G in cases in which the oral route is desirable, but it is less effective than penicillin G against gram-negative microorganisms, especially *Neisseria* species. (Thus, it is not recommended for gonococcal infections.) Like penicillin G, this agent is not effective against penicillinase-producing bacteria.

INDICATIONS	Penicillin V potassium is indicated in the treatment of mild to moderately severe infections due to penicillin G-sensitive microorganisms. This drug is indicated for mild to moderate streptococcal infections of the upper respiratory tract, scarlet fever, and mild erysipelas; mild to moderate pneumococcal infections of the respiratory tract; mild penicillin G-sensitive staphylococcal infections of the skin and soft tissues. (Reports indicate an increasing number of resistant strains.) Infections of the oropharynx, mild to moderate, due to Fusospirochetes (Vincent's gingivitis and pharyngitis) usually respond. It is indicated for the prevention of recurrence following rheumatic fever and/or chorea and for prevention of infections in certain cardiac patients undergoing dental procedures or minor upper respiratory tract surgery or instrumentation. Prophylaxis should be started on the day of the procedure and continued for 2 or more days following.
PREPARATIONS	Tablets: 125, 250, or 500 mg (equivalent to 200,000, 400,000, or 800,000 units of penicillin V, respectively). Oral solution: 125 or 250 mg per 5 ml of solution (teaspoon).
DOSAGE	The usual adult oral dosage range is 125–500 mg four to six times daily. The usual oral dosage range in children is 25–50 mg/kg body weight daily administered in divided doses every 6–8 hours. For prophylactic treatment of rheumatic fever in adults, 125–250 mg daily.
CONTRAINDICATIONS AND PRECAUTIONS	Known hypersensitivity to penicillins is a contraindication; use cautiously in patients with allergies and/or asthma.
ADVERSE REACTIONS	Hypersensitivity reactions are fairly com-

mon (1–5%), gastrointestinal reactions occur, and superinfections with resistant organisms (such as gram-negative bacteria) can occur. Blood dyscrasias, neuropathy, and nephropathy occur rarely and are usually associated with high doses of parenteral penicillin. The penicillins are otherwise essentially nontoxic in man. Among 707 patients on penicillin VK studied in the Boston Collaborative Drug Surveillance Program 19 patients had side effects as follows: sensitivity reactions (10), gastrointestinal disturbances (6), and "other" (3).

LITERATURE

AMA Drug Evaluations, 4th ed. New York, AMA and Wiley, 1980, Chapter 69; Mandell, GL, Sande, MA: In The Pharmacological Basis of Therapeutics, 6th ed (Gilman, AG, Goodman, LS, Gilman, A, eds). New York, Macmillan, 1980, Chapter 50; Medical Letter 24:21, 1982 (choice of antimicrobials).

VIBRAMYCIN® (Pfizer)
Doxycycline (hyclate, calcium, or monohydrate)

1981:68
1980:49
1979:48

Doxycycline, one of the tetracyclines, is synthetically derived from oxytetracycline. It has the same broad-spectrum antimicrobial activity as that of other tetracyclines. It is superior to other analogues, however, in that it has excellent absorption following oral administration and a longer serum half-life than most other tetracyclines.

INDICATIONS

Tetracyclines are indicated in infections caused by the following: Rickettsiae, *Mycoplasma pneumonia*, agents of psittacosis and ornithosis, agents of lymphogranuloma

336

venereum and granuloma inguinale, and the spirochetal agent of relapsing fever (*Borrelia recurrentis*). The following gram-negative microorganisms are also sensitive: *Haemophilus ducreyi*, *Pasteurella* species, *Bartonella bacilliformis*, *Bacteroides* species, *Vibrio comma* and *Vibrio fetus* and *Brucella* species (in conjunction with streptomycin). *Tetracyclines* are alternates to penicillin in treating infections due to: *Neisseria gonorrhea*, *Treponema pallidum* and *Treponema pertenue*, *Listeria*, *Clostridium*, *Bacillus anthracis*, *Fusobacterium fusiforme* (Vincent's infection) and *Actinomyces* species. Certain other gram-positive and gram-negative microorganisms may be treated with tetracyclines when bacteriologic testing indicates appropriate susceptibility. *Tetracyclines* are usually not useful in streptococcal diseases; they have been successfully used in the management of acne. Other indications are in the treatment of trachoma and in inclusion conjunctivitis.

PREPARATIONS

Capsules (doxycycline hyclate): 50 and 100 mg. Tablets (Vibra-Tabs) (doxycycline hyclate): 100 mg. Oral suspension (doxycycline calcium): each 5 ml (teaspoon) contains 50 mg. Oral suspension (doxycycline monohydrate): each 5 ml (teaspoon), when reconstituted, contains 25 mg.

DOSAGE

Adults: 100 mg *orally* at 12 hour intervals for two doses, followed by 100 mg once daily as a single dose or as 50 mg every 12 hrs. For severe infections, 100 mg every 12 hours may be continued. When the intravenous route is used the initial dose is 200 mg on the first day given in one or two infusions, followed by 100–200 mg daily. Children above 8 years: the recommended dose in children weighing 100

337

lbs or less is 2 mg/lb divided into 2 doses on the first day, followed by 1 mg/lb given as a single daily dose or divided into two doses on subsequent days. For more severe infections up to 2 mg/lb may be used.

For syphilis, 300 mg daily (orally) in divided doses for at least 10 days. Acute gonococcal infections require 200 mg stat and 100 mg at bedtime the first day (orally), followed by 100 mg b.i.d. for 3 days.

Note: *The usual dosage schedule of doxycycline differs from that of the other tetracyclines.*

CONTRAINDICATIONS AND PRECAUTIONS

This drug is contraindicated in persons who have shown hypersensitivity to any of the tetracyclines. Use of tetracyclines during tooth development may cause permanent discoloration of the teeth. Use with caution in the presence of hepatic or renal impairment. Photosensitivity may be induced by tetracyclines. Prolonged use may lead to superinfection. Safety during pregnancy and nursing, or in the newborn, has not been established.

ADVERSE REACTIONS

Gastrointestinal disturbances (nausea and vomiting) are the most common adverse effects; tooth discoloration (as described above) can occur. Less frequent adverse reactions include malabsorption, enterocolitis, photosensitivity, and various sensitivity reactions. Superinfection, rise in BUN, and renal damage may occur. Other reactions occur, but are rare. Among 1172 patients on tetracyclines studied in the Boston Collaborative Drug Surveillance Program 73 patients had adverse reactions as follows: gastrointestinal disturbances (41), superinfection (9), rise in BUN (8), sensitivity reactions (8), injection site complications (5), and "other" (2). These drugs interact with oral antacids, bismuth subsalicylate, oral contraceptives, oral iron, methoxyflurane, and zinc sulfate. This drug seems to cause more transient reversible vestibular reactions than other tetracyclines. Tetracyclines have been shown to depress plasma prothrombin activity. Patients on anticoagulants may require lower doses of the anticoagulant.

LITERATURE   Am Acad Dermatol (Ad Hoc Committee on Antibiotics): Arch Dermatol 111:1630, 1975; Finland, M: Clin Pharmacol Ther 15:3, 1974 (commentary on tetracyclines); Johnson, AH: Semin Drug Treat 2:331, 1972 (adverse effects); Medical Letter 24:21, 1982 (choice of antimicrobials); Sack, DA, et al: N Engl J Med 298:758, 1978 (travelers' diarrhea); Siegel, D: NY State J Med 78:950 and 1115, 1978 (reviews on tetracyclines).

VIBRA-TABS® (Pfizer)
Doxycycline hyclate

1981:172
1980: —
1979: —

This preparation is available as film coated tablets containing doxycycline hyclate equivalent to 100 mg of doxycycline. For further information, see VIBRAMYCIN.

VISTARIL® (Pfizer)
Hydroxyzine pamoate

1981:166
1980:152
1979:156

Vistaril is broadly classified as a tranquilizer. It is not chemically related to the phenothiazines, reserpine, or meprobamate. Hydroxyzine has been shown clinically to be a rapid-acting ataraxic. It is not a cortical depressant, but its action may be due to suppression of its activity in certain key regions in the subcortical area of the central nervous system. Experimentally, hydroxyzine has been shown to have antispasmodic properties apparently mediated through interference with the mechanism that responds to spasmogenic agents such as serotonin, acetylcholine, and histamine. It also has antihistaminic effects and a possible antiemetic effect.

INDICATIONS

Vistaril is indicated for symptomatic relief of anxiety and tension associated with psychoneurosis and as an adjunct in organic states in which anxiety is manifested. It is also used in the management of pruritus due to allergic conditions such as chronic urticaria and atopic and contact dermatoses, and in histamine-mediated pruritis. Vistaril is also used as a sedative for premedication and following general anesthesia. Hydroxyzine may potentiate meperidine and barbiturates.

PREPARATIONS

Capsules (hydroxyzine pamoate equivalent to hydroxyzine hydrochloride): 25, 50 and 100 mg. Suspension: equivalent to 25 mg hydroxyzine HCl per 5 ml.

DOSAGE

For anxiety in adults: 50–100 mg four times a day. Children over 6 years: 50–100 mg daily in divided doses; children under 6 years: 50 mg daily in divided doses. For pruritis the usual adult dose is 25 mg three or four times per day, whereas the dose in children is as follows: 50–100 mg daily (divided doses) for children over 6 years and 50 mg daily (divided) for children under 6 years. When used as a sedative for premedication and following general anesthesia the adult dose is 50–100 mg and the child's dose is 0.6 mg/kg.

CONTRAINDICATIONS
AND PRECAUTIONS

Hydroxyzine is contraindicated in early pregnancy and in nursing mothers. It is also contraindicated in patients with previous demonstration of hypersensitivity to the drug.

ADVERSE REACTIONS

Side effects reported with recommended doses of Vistaril are mild and transitory in nature. These are dry mouth, drowsiness, and involuntary motor activity. The Boston Collaborative Drug Surveillance Program study found these mild side effects occurred in only 3 of 137 patients studied. Hydroxyzine may potentiate meperidine (Demerol®) and barbiturates.

LITERATURE

Baraf, CS: Curr Ther Res 19:32, 1976; Barranco, SF, Bridger, W: Curr Ther Res 22:217, 1977; Dilts, SL, et al: Am J Psychiat 134:92, 1977; Massound, N: J Pediatr 93:308, 1978; Rhoades, RB, et al: J Allergy Clin Immunol 55:180, 1975; Tobias, M, et al: J Dent Child 42:453, 1975.

ZAROXOLYN® (Pennwalt)
Metolazone

1981:152
1980:172
1979:185

Metolazone, a sulfonamide diuretic antihypertensive agent, has pharmacologic properties similar to the thiazide diuretics. It acts primarily to inhibit sodium reabsorption at the cortical diluting site and in the proximal convoluted tubule. Sodium and chloride ions are excreted at approximately equivalent amounts.

INDICATIONS

Zaroxolyn is indicated in the management of hypertension either as the sole therapeutic agent or to enhance the effectiveness of other antihypertensive drugs. It is also used for the treatment of salt and

341

water retention in congestive heart failure and in renal diseases.

PREPARATIONS

Tablets: 2.5, 5, and 10 mg.

DOSAGE

The dosage must be individualized to the patient and the severity of the condition. Usual ranges are as follows: *Edema of cardiac failure:* 5–10 mg once daily; *edema of renal disease:* 5–20 mg once daily; mild to moderate essential hypertension, 2.5–5 mg once daily. Zaroxolyn is a potent drug with a prolonged, 12–24 hour duration of action.

CONTRAINDICATIONS AND PRECAUTIONS

This drug is contraindicated in individuals with a known hypersensitivity to metolazone and in patients with anuria, hepatic coma, or precoma. All patients receiving Zaroxolyn therapy should be observed for electrolyte imbalance (see product insert for details). Safety for use during pregnancy, nursing, or in children has not been established.

ADVERSE REACTIONS

Hypokalemia, hyperglycemia, hyponatremia, hypochloremia, hyperuricemia, and glycosuria can occur. Gastrointestinal disturbances, CNS reactions (dizziness, vertigo, paresthesias, headache, syncope, and drowsiness), hematologic reactions, and hypersensitivity dermatologic reactions can occur. Orthostatic hypotension may also occur with this drug. Acute gouty attacks, chills, muscle cramps or spasm, increase in BUN, and restlessness have occurred. Adverse effects and drug interactions are generally similar to those of thiazides.

LITERATURE

Fotiu, S, et al: Clin Pharmacol Ther 16:318, 1974; Pilewski, RM, et al: Clin Pharmacol Ther 12:843, 1971. See also Medical Letter 21:40, 1979, for further

discussion of metolazone and Medical
Letter 23:45, 1981 for a review on drugs
for hypertension.

ZOMAX® (McNeil)
Zomepirac sodium

1981:54
1980:—
1979:—

Zomepirac is a new nonsteroidal anti-inflammatory analgesic that
is chemically related to tolmetin; it is an inhibitor of prostaglandin
synthetase. Clinical trials have shown that zomepirac is a potent
and effective analgesic, more effective than aspirin, and possibly preferable to oral narcotics for moderate pain (not relieved by aspirin)
since there is no apparent tolerance or potential for addiction. This
compound is not a substitute for parenteral morphine in the treatment of severe pain.

INDICATIONS	Zomax is indicated for the relief of mild to moderately severe pain.
PREPARATIONS	Tablets: 100 mg.
DOSAGE	The recommended dosage is 100 mg every 4 to 6 hrs as required. In mild pain 50 mg every 4 to 6 hrs may be adequate. (Doses exceeding 600 mg per day are not recommended.)
CONTRAINDICATIONS AND PRECAUTIONS	Zomax should not be used in patients who have previously exhibited tolerance to it nor should it be used in patients in whom aspirin or other nonsteroidal anti-inflammatory drugs induce bronchospasm, rhinitis, or urticaria. Concomitant use with aspirin is not recommended. Zomax is not recommended in children, in pregnant women, or in nursing mothers.
ADVERSE REACTIONS	The most frequent adverse reaction is nausea which occurred in 12% of patients

during clinical trials (6% in short-term therapy). Other gastrointestinal reactions with a frequency of 3 to 9% were: gastrointestinal distress, diarrhea, abdominal pain, dyspepsia, constipation, flatulence and vomiting. Gastritis and anorexia occurred less frequently. Other reactions occurring in 3 to 9% of patients were: dizziness, insomnia, edema, elevation in blood pressure, rash, asthenia, and urinary tract infection. Other CNS, cardiovascular, psychiatric, urogenital, dermatologic and gastrointestinal effects occurred less frequently. Tinnitus and change in taste were also reported.

LITERATURE

Medical Letter 23:1, 1981 (review with additional references).

ZYLOPRIM® (Burroughs Wellcome)
Allopurinol

1981:56
1980:59
1979:59

Allopurinol is effective for the therapy of both the primary hyperuricemia of gout and that secondary to other conditions. It blocks the terminal steps in uric acid biosynthesis by inhibition of xanthine oxidase.

INDICATIONS

Zyloprim is intended for the treatment of gout, either primary or secondary to the hyperuricemia associated with blood diseases and the therapy of those diseases. It is also used in the treatment of primary or secondary uric acid nephropathy, with or without accompanying symptoms of gout. It is used in patients with recurrent uric acid stone formation and as a prophylactic agent in the treatment to prevent

344

tissue urate disposition, renal calculi, or uric acid nephropathy in patients receiving cancer chemotherapy.

PREPARATIONS

Tablets: 100 and 300 mg.

DOSAGE

For treating gout and to lower serum uric acid the dosage depends on the severity of the disease. For mild gout, 200–300 mg per day; for moderately severe tophaceous gout, 400–600 mg per day. (Dosages less than 300 mg may be administered divided or as a single dose.) For prevention of uric acid nephropathy during treatment of neoplastic disease, 600–800 mg daily for 2 or 3 days together with a high fluid intake. (See package insert for futher details on dosages.)

CONTRAINDICATIONS AND PRECAUTIONS

Zyloprim is contraindicated in nursing mothers and in children, with the exception of children with hyperuricemia secondary to malignancy. Patients who have had a severe reaction should not be restarted on the drug. Zyloprim should be discontinued at the first sign of skin rash or any sign of adverse reaction. Use with caution in patients with preexisting liver or kidney disease. Zyloprim administered concomitantly with Purinethol (mercaptopurine) or Imuran (azathioprine) will require subsequent reduction in the dosage of Purinethol or Imuran. Safety for use in pregnancy and in women of childbearing age has not been established.

ADVERSE REACTIONS

Sensitivity reactions are the most common; hematologic and gastrointestinal disturbances also occur. Less frequently seen are hepatic, vascular, renal, neurologic, and ophthalmic reactions. Among 938 patients on allopurinol studied in the Boston Collaborative Drug Surveillance Program 33 patients had side effects as follows: sensitivity reactions (rash or drug fever) (21), hematologic complications (thrombocytopenia, leukopenia) (6), gastrointestinal disturbances (3), and "other" (3). Allopurinal interacts with oral anticoagulants, azathioprine, cyclophosphamide, and mercaptopurine.

LITERATURE

Elion, GB: In Uric Acid: Handbook of Experimental Pharmacology (Kelley, WN, Weiner, IM, eds). Berlin, Springer-Verlag, 1978, Chapter 21.

346